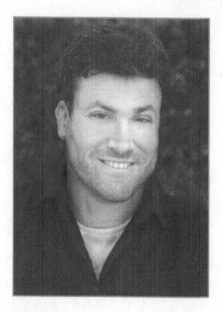

About the Author

Greg Wolfe grew up in Southern California and attended UC Santa Barbara and UC San Diego. After college, he studied comedy writing and performing with the Ground-lings and ACME Theater improv groups in Los Angeles while earning his master's degree in education. He now teaches high school English and history. Currently resid-ing in Valencia, California, Greg and his wife, Julie (a TV and film writer), went through four IVF cycles before joy-fully welcoming their son, Connor, into the world in March 2009. Connor owes them big-time.

HARPER

NEW YORK • LONDON • TORONTO • SYDNEY

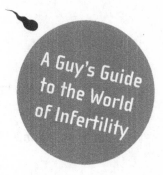

A Guy's Guide
to the World
of Infertility

How to Make

Love

to a

PLASTIC
CUP

GREG WOLFE

To Julie and Connor,
for making each day
seem better than the last.
I love you both more
than you'll ever know.

HARPER

HarperCollins books may be purchased for educational, business, or sales promotional use. For information please, e-mail the Special Markets Department at SPsales@harpercollins.com.

FIRST EDITION

Designed by Janet M. Evans

Library of Congress Cataloging-in-Publication data is available upon request.

ISBN 978-0-06-185948-9

17 18 19 OV/RRD 10 9 8 7 6 5 4 3 2

CONTENTS

FOREWORD

Men deal with problems differently than women, a fact that dates all the way back to Adam and Eve in the Garden of Eden. While both Adam and Eve ate the fruit of knowledge, it was Eve who asked the serpent some questions first, whereas Adam simply took it from her on good faith. This is not to say that men are more superficial or ignorant than women. They simply believe that asking questions shows weakness. That is why they don't like asking for directions, but will gladly use their GPS.

This guy's guide is a GPS for dealing with infertility. Now you, the reader, can secretly peek into it anytime your wife or doctor uses this foreign language called "fertilitish," and you'll not only understand every word and nuance, but you might even surprise them from time to time with some coherent feedback.

I cannot think of a more qualified person to write a book about fertility treatment from a guy's point of view than Greg, a seasoned veteran of the fertility struggle, one who has experienced firsthand and in a most courageous and selfless manner the grinding daily burden and sacrifice that pave the way to victory (i.e., a baby).

My first encounter with Greg and Julie in 2008 was not unlike many other consultations I have had with infertile patients over the past twenty-three years. In the course of such consultations, I usually scan dozens of pages of medical records relating to prior failed therapies in an attempt to plan the best treatment strategy. In contrast to many other husbands, however, Greg demonstrated a depth of knowledge and involvement in Julie's treatment, which ultimately contributed to their success. During one of our long conversations, he mentioned his intent to write a fertility guide for men after the successful completion of the treatment.

Amazingly, Greg managed to complete both "projects"—his son Connor and this book—in the most wonderful fashion. Regretfully, Connor—as gorgeous as he is—can only be enjoyed by Greg, Julie, and a few others. This book, on the other hand, is available for the benefit of all humanity, and I think they're going to love it. It successfully conveys the information while being extremely funny. The choice of metaphors and analogies from a guy's realm is nothing short of genius, yet through it all Greg maintains an impressive level of medical accuracy. In other words, this is the ultimate guy's GPS to fertility, narrated by a comedian. I will undoubtedly hand it to my patients.

Michael Vermesh, M.D.
Associate Professor, USC
Center for Fertility and Gynecology
Tarzana, California
October 2009

AUTHOR'S NOTE

This book should not be considered a substitute for professional medical advice; for more information, consult your
own reproductive medical professional. Although this book
is a good general look at the various infertility treatments
available, by no means should the information herein be considered a "blanket standard," as each couple's experiences
will be different. I need to seriously stress here that I'm not a
doctor. Nor have I even set foot in a medical school. Heck, I
don't even look that good in the color green.

INTRODUCTION

Since before recorded time, no matter the species, males have been programmed with one biological imperative, one need above all others—the need to reproduce. From the time the first multicelled organism crawled its way out of the primordial soup and thought to itself, "Gee, I wish I had a smaller version of me to play ball with," men have wanted to have children.

Even today, with the advent of the 54" LCD TV and 5.1 THX-equipped home theater systems, procreating still ranks pretty darn high up on our list.

For some of us, it's all about continuing the family name. For others, it's about leaving a legacy in this world that will endure long after we're gone. Or hey, maybe you just want someone to help with the yard work. Regardless of the reason, once we get the idea in our heads to be a daddy, there's nothing we won't endure in order to reproduce.

Think of all the things you went through—nights out at bars, meeting women at parties, horrible blind dates, unreturned phone calls, crazy stalkers with unresolved "daddy issues"—all of those ordeals that you had to withstand in the hopes of finding that special someone, your perfect match, with whom you wanted to 1) settle down, and 2) raise a family.

For the purposes of this book, I'll assume you already have number one covered. As the ancient Babylonians used to say, "Mazel tov!" It's hard enough to find someone who can put up with your day-to-day bathroom habits, let alone be your soul mate, so consider that a huge accomplishment unto itself. Now as for number two—well, that may be a bit more complicated . . .

———

When my wife, Julie, and I got married in 2002, we were a couple of young crazy kids (well, thirty—but still crazy) and felt that even though a family was definitely in our future, it might be fun just to be a couple for a while. Plus, we lived in Hollywood, and we wanted nothing more than to experience the cool, hip L.A. lifestyle: drink and eat at all the fabulous new bars and restaurants that are always popping up around town, check out art shows at the local galleries, etc. Then, eventually, when we were burnt out on being social butterflies, we'd do the "family thing." And we did just that.

Well, when I say "that," I mean we sat around our apartment, had pizza delivered, and drank Two Buck Chuck while we watched TV. Yeah, it turns out we weren't quite as young and hip as we thought we were. Clubs are open really late, you know? So one day, during a commercial break, we looked at one another and said, "Maybe now would be a good time to pull that 'having a family' idea out of the mothballs."

Thus we came to the momentous decision that it was time to have children. Of course we made a big deal about it to our family and friends. "So, you ready to be grandparents?" "Hey, can we count on you to babysit?" "Hope your sofa is vomit-proof!" And then we tried. And tried. And tried. For a whole year. Then two.

Now the pesky little problem with being all cocky and telling people you're going to do something as momentous as reproducing is that, well, they actually expect results. So the private anguish that Julie and I were going through was compounded tenfold by the constant questions about our progress: "What? You're *still* not pregnant?" "Hey, we Scotch-guarded our sofa and everything—so where the hell's the baby?" "Wow, are you two even trying?"

Were we trying? Um, *yeah*. You know that annoying-as-crap couple who look at each other lovingly, squeeze each other's hand, smile, and say, "I don't know. We just tried once and boom!" followed by peals of smug laughter? I hate those people. Figuring we were just one of the other kinds of couples—the unlucky ones who have to try a little harder—we tried a little harder. And we waited. And waited. And—well, you get the running joke here. Until eventually we started thinking that maybe, just maybe, something was wrong. And unfortunately, we found out that we were right . . .

———

Infertility has increased significantly as a problem over the last thirty years. According to the 2002 National Survey of Family Growth by the CDC:

- Of the approximately 62 million women of reproductive age in 2002, about 1.2 million, or 2 percent, had had an infertility-related medical appointment within the previous year and an additional 10 percent had received infertility services at some time in their lives. (Infertility services include medical tests to diagnose infertility, medical advice and treatments like in vitro fertilization to help a woman become pregnant, and services other than routine prenatal care to prevent miscarriage.)

- Additionally, 7 percent of married couples in which the woman was of reproductive age (2.1 million couples) reported that they had not used contraception for twelve months and the woman had not become pregnant.[a]

What does all that mean? It means you aren't alone. Millions of people are going through the exact same things as you are, and dealing with exactly the same problems. It's a small comfort, but it's a comfort.

Now, if you're like most men, right about now you're probably asking, "Huh? What's in vitro? Oh, wait—isn't that the thing where we get to mix up our kid in a beaker? Cool! I'll take mine with blond hair and a wicked good change-up pitch!" That's right. We're dumb.

Oh, our wives know all about it (infertility, I mean—not about us being dumb—though I think they may be getting suspicious). After all, they've spent days and weeks endlessly researching the subject, buying up every book they can find, carefully screening fertility doctors, and lurking around the dozens of online message boards devoted to the subject. We men, however, have kind of been given short shrift.

When we began going through infertility treatments, we found loads of books, but all of them seemed geared directly toward women—specifically, women who have a lot of time to read. Seriously, I had college textbooks that were less dense. And what's with the names? They're all so soft and, well, fluffy: *Your Infertility and You, Two Can Be the Loneliest Number, Mommy and (Not) Me,* and on and on. I dutifully tried flipping through them, but they were obviously for women's eyes only. Kind of like the Lifetime channel.

Oh, sure, maybe there were one or two throwaway chapters for us men; we got a few crumbs of info, but nothing particularly helpful or informative: "Sperm helps makes babies," "This is a penis. You have one"—that sort of thing. Personally, I found it kind of irritating. I mean we're worth twenty-three out of forty-six chromosomes. Shouldn't we be allowed a little insight and information on the process too? I say, "Yes, dammit!"

Well take heart, because this book you so wisely bought (okay, more likely that your wife bought for you) will help guide you, the man, through all the highs and lows, the yin and the yang of the myriad of available infertility treatments and how they work. We're talking the whole gamut of biology, from soup to, er . . . nuts. Most importantly, you'll find out what *your* part will be in the process.

Even if you don't know the difference between IUI and IVF, or can't tell a test tube from a fallopian tube, by the time you're done here you're sure to feel a lot more confident in knowing what you're doing. Plus your wife will be incredibly impressed and you'll be her hero. And at the end of the day, isn't that really what we all want?

Well, that and the 54" LCD TV.

ONE

Begin by Putting Tab "A" into Slot "B"

*M*ost of the time, it's an easy enough recipe: Take one man, add one woman, shake vigorously, let sit for nine months, and voilà! "Here's your baby, be sure to hold it with both hands, don't forget to feed it, etc." Piece of cake, right? Hell, it seems like for some guys—usually greasy-haired-backward-baseball-cap-wearing dirtbags married to pop singers—they just have to *look* at a woman and she's pregnant. But the sad truth is that it's not always as easy to conceive as those irresponsible, wacky celebrities on TMZ make it look.

For Julie and me, deciding to put off starting a family didn't mean that we didn't want kids—far from it. We were both raised in very close, loving (if not slightly neurotic) families, and we were excited about the idea of someday starting a slightly less neurotic family of our own. (You always want your kids to do better than you did.)

At that particular moment in time, however, we felt that we still had lots of important things to do first: What with our burgeoning careers, active social lives, and spur-of-the-moment trips to Vegas, we were swamped. Besides . . . we had *plenty* of time.

You're probably thinking, "Greg, you selfish bastard! Only thinking about yourself and whether or not you should double down with a soft fourteen against the dealer's four!" But in all fairness, I had lots of love to share, Julie too. And share the love we did—with our four cats.

Yes, a man can love cats. Shut up.

Plus, I'm a high school teacher, so I already have the . . . um . . . *pleasure* of dealing with 180 teenagers, six hours a day. For those that haven't heard about the schools in California, let's just say they're not exactly advertisements for the joys of reproduction. I'm not saying that all teenagers are bad. Wait, yes, yes I am. They're awful. And from all accounts a vaccine is still years away . . .

Time passed, and at last, the momentous time had arrived. Julie and I were ready to spawn. We decided to make the night special. We were actually so cute and naïve as to think we could pick the night of conception. We did the whole "romantic dinner, back to the apartment and have a nightcap" thing, and then, just like Babe Ruth calling his shot, we went for it.

Oddly enough, we didn't get pregnant immediately. "Oh, well," we thought, "who gets pregnant on the first try?" So we figured we'd try again. "Hey, practice makes perfect, right?" we laughed, oh so charmingly, while clinking our martini glasses and listening to smooth jazz (okay, not really, but it sounds classy, right?).

After many months of trying, I have to admit that I was beginning to get slightly . . . peeved. Julie and I had segued from romantic lovemaking between a husband and wife into a highly structured time, temperature, and pee-stick-specific breeding regimen. By means of comparison, think of your favorite burger. Yum. Now, think of being told you have to eat it a certain way. And furthermore, you *have* to eat it whenever it reaches a certain temperature outside, whether you're hungry or not. I'm not quite sure where the pee stick fits into this metaphor, but you get the general idea.

And as the months went by, that which I thought could never happen, happened: Sex became a chore, like doing laundry or grouting the tub. I wasn't the only one who felt it. Julie's signals to retire to the bedroom went from a coy "Shall we go to bed?" smile to an "Okay, fine, let's do this" sigh. Nevertheless, we were still committed to having a baby. I was going to have someone to teach how to tie his teeny tiny Keds or die trying, dammit!

After many unsuccessful months of appointment sex—and then weeks more of Googling dozens of fertility Web sites—Julie gently suggested that maybe we might need some help, that this process might require, well, someone more than just the two of us.

Naturally, I was thrilled by the idea—until I realized that she meant seeing a fertility specialist.

LOOK, IT'S NOT YOU, IT'S ME

At the risk of sounding all Tim Allen here, we men do not like anyone telling us that we can't fix something ourselves. I don't care if it's a $10,000 supercomputer with state-of-the-art bioorganic motherboards; if it's on the fritz, just hand us a claw hammer and stand back. So the thought that something might be wrong with us—like, *really* wrong—didn't sit well with me. I mean, how hard can it be? There are kids all over the place! So why the hell were we having so much trouble? Even worse was when, after a slew of tests, we found out that, as the old line goes, "It's not her; it's me."

Yep, turns out I was low in almost every possible sperm measurement—quantity, quality, and movement. (I was probably deficient in "color," "cut," and "clarity" too, but I couldn't bear to look at the rest of the lab report.) Basically, my sperm wouldn't be able to find its way to Julie's eggs if it had a Triple-A TripTik and a GPS system. *Wow.* Talk about taking the wind out of your sails.

But when you want a child as badly as we did, you don't let a little thing like the complete decimation of everything that it means to be a man stop you. So, after I carefully packed my battered male ego into a little box to be opened during future therapy sessions, Julie and I talked at length with our doctor about our options, and together we all set off down that long, unpaved, and winding path known as "fertility treatments."

Julie had done all of the research, of course. She signed up for all of the Web sites and message boards, and by the time our doctor laid out our options, she was ready. She asked intelligent questions; he nodded and gave intelligent answers. I suppose. I say "I suppose" because I had *no frigging idea* what they were talking about. I admit it. I didn't study for the test, and it showed.

In order to figure out and understand what your specific fertility problem is, and what treatment will work best for you, you need to go back to the beginning and learn a few things. Actually, a lot of things. But as the saying goes, you can't put up a skyscraper without a solid foundation, so the first thing you need is a little refresher course on basic human biology, conveniently found in the next chapter. Oh come on, read it. It has the words "penis" and "vagina" in there a bunch of times . . .

TWO

Basic Biology for
Complete and
Utter Dummies
(No Offense)

So, ready for a test? Okay, pencils up . . . what do you remember from high school biology?

No, I don't mean playing paper football in the back row or drawing on your Pee Chee folder so that one basketball player looked like he was stabbing the other one or "accidentally" dropping your pen so you could get a quick look at Abby Bettencourt's legs on those Fridays when she wore her cheerleader outfit. I mean what do you remember about *biology*? You know: genetics, Punnett squares, reproduction? All that boring stuff?

Well, if you're trying to have a child, especially through infertility treatments, you'd better remember, and fast. Over the coming days, weeks, and months you'll be hearing so much about zygotes, blastocysts, ova, spermatozoa, etc., that you'll want to pull off your own ears and give 'em to the dogs as chew toys. Face it. You need a refresher course.

Not to say that you don't know the basics. I hope. I mean it's all fine and dandy to say that the penis goes into the vagina and a baby comes out. Great. My six-year-old nephew knows that. Yeah, we all know that it takes a sperm and an egg to make a baby, but how exactly does it happen? Where do they come from? How do they meet? Once they get together, what do they talk about? These are things you really should know, not only to help you through these infertility processes, but also so you don't look like a complete schmuck.

So let's take things one step at a time, and start with your junk.

MAN, IT'S HARDER THAN CALCULUS

Now when most men are asked about their reproductive system, they think of their penises. For that matter, when most men are asked about the electric bill, their favorite movie, or if they had a good weekend they think of their penises. We're very focused in that way. That's okay though: It's the human male's incessant thought, need, and drive for sex that has allowed us to flourish as a species—and kept booze companies in business for centuries to boot. Except for Zima. Nobody liked Zima.

Looking at the penis itself, it's not particularly impressive. That's not a slight on you; it's just a general truth. After all, it's basically just a tube made up of two different kinds of tissue: spongy and cartilaginous, all surrounded by very sensitive skin.

Now normally, it just hangs there, quietly, just trying to stay out of the way of stray kicks and zippers and things. But when you see something arousing, or think about something arousing, or, hey, for a lot of us, when you're just sitting there balancing out the accounts receivable ledger, the floodgates open up, and the blood starts flowing—actually *blasting*—under extremely high pressure, down into your little soldier. It fills up all of the spaces in the hard cartilage tissue and then becomes trapped in there, which, ultimately, serves to make you, well, hard. Good to go. Ready for business.

When you're finished (or when your boss suddenly comes into your office), the same valves that snapped shut to trap all that blood in your penis in the first place relax, which allows the blood to flow out again, returning you to your normal flaccid state.

But the thing to remember is that although the penis is a great delivery system, there is more—much more—to the male reproductive system than the penis. It's like looking at a light bulb and saying that's where electricity comes from. No sir, what we need to do is go a bit deeper inside and see what all you've got going on in there.

YOU MUST BE NUTS

A lot of guys think their testicles are like the fuzzy dice hanging from a car's rearview mirror: Sure they look cool and maybe they're fun to play with occasionally, but they don't make or break the car. Wrong. When it comes to baby making, your testicles are the A-number-one most important weapons in your arsenal. Another difference is that if you accidentally hit the fuzzy dice, your car doesn't scream, curl up into a ball, and throw up nonstop.

Your testicles are where your spermatozoa, or the male sex cell, is created and stored. That's the reason they hang away from your body: The sperm requires lower than body temperature to survive, so the separation acts as a kind of refrigeration system.

Because of this, there is more than a little bit of truth to the whole "don't wear tight underwear" old wives' tale. If your scrotum is pressed against your body, it heats up and wham: sperm soup. The same goes for hot baths, hot tubs, and Jacuzzis. You boil your boys too much, and nothing's coming out of there alive.

Now for what's inside. A lot of men, and quite a few women, equate sperm—which, as I said, is the male sex cell—with semen, which is the fluid that contains the sperm. As a result, guys figure that when they ejaculate they need to gush like a porn star. But the truth is that isn't the truth. A man can produce a large amount of semen with very few sperm, or they can have a vast number of sperm in relatively little semen. We'll talk sperm in greater detail later, but first let's take a look at semen.

SAY IT, DON'T SPRAY IT

The fluid that makes up semen comes from three different glands: the Cowper's gland, the seminal vesicles, and the prostate gland. "Uh, what?" I hear you say. Each gland adds something different to the mix, so all three are equally important when it comes to making your semen. Let me break it down for you:

The Cowper's gland is actually a pair of glands at the base of the penis. During sexual arousal, their job is to create a thick fluid (called *pre-ejaculate*) that neutralizes any acidic urine that may still be hanging around in your urethra. This fluid, which makes up around 10–15 percent of your semen, also acts as a really slippery lubricant, turning your urethra into a giant Slip 'n Slide for your sperm. It may also carry any leftover sperm from your last ejaculation, which is the reason you were always told that you could still get a girl pregnant having unprotected sex even if you don't ejaculate in her—although, if you're reading this now, I'm guessing that's not such a big concern for you at the moment.

The seminal vesicles are perched on top of your prostate gland, and are responsible for making the seminal fluid, which constitutes 60 percent of your semen. They also make the semen slightly alkaline, which is necessary in order for the sperm to survive in the vagina (see below).

The prostate gland is most generally talked about later in a man's life, as in, "Oy vey! My doctor just told me that my prostate is the size of a Valencia orange!" But it's much more than a funny complaint. In fact, it is a crucial part of a man's reproductive system, as the fluid it produces makes up the remaining 25–30 percent of your semen. The sperm that come out bathed in this prostatic fluid are better protected, survive longer, and move better than those just swimming around in the seminal fluid alone.

When the actual sperm cells—the little wriggly things that actually go into the egg and make a baby—are shuttled from your testicles through a tube called the *vas deferens*, they are bathed in the combination of all these various fluids we just talked about, and bam: There's your semen!

Even though, at the end of the day, it's the sperm that gets the job done and thus gets all the accolades, the little-considered semen that has been combined from all your glands is incredibly important for the number of things that it does to make insemination possible—not to mention it's actually really neat:

1. It works as both a transport medium and an energy source for your sperm, acting like a liquefied Clif Bar, feeding them enough so they can wiggle those little tails all the way to the finish of their "swim of love."

2. It neutralizes the acid in the vagina (yes, a woman's vagina is filled with acid—deal with it). Actually, we'll get to that in a second, so don't panic or make a grossed-out face, because if your wife is in the room she'll look at you funny and ask what's wrong and you'll have to tell her and she'll get all defensive about her acidic vagina and that's a whole headache you don't need.

3. It contains a chemical that causes the woman's uterus to contract, which aids in pushing the sperm upward and onward toward its goal.

See? I told you it was neat. And here you thought it was only good for starching your socks.

Now, as I mentioned before, a great deal of semen doesn't necessarily mean there's a great deal of sperm. In fact, of the total content of the semen, only 1 percent is actually sperm, which is why more often it's quality, and not quantity, that matters when talking about making babies.

WHEN IT COMES TO WOMEN, IT'S WHAT'S INSIDE THAT COUNTS

Okay, now it's time to get down and dirty, and move to the thing that every guy thinks he's an expert in, but in reality has no idea about. I refer, of course, to the female reproductive system.

To start with, you may have noticed in the midst of your lifelong trials and tribulations with the opposite sex that with women everything is hidden inside, nice and neatly tucked away, as opposed to us men with our big swinging penises and dangling scrotums. Ugh. It's a wonder any woman would have us at all.

Okay, now you're about to get smart. Did you know that there's a biological and a sociological reason we men are all out there and dangly? It's because, as with all males in the animal kingdom, nature has declared that we have to do the attracting in whatever courtship rituals we practice, in order to get the females to want to mate with us. Moreover, we must convince the females that our genes are superior to another competing male's. Different animals do it differently: Baboons compare who has the biggest, reddest ass. Mountain goats run around ramming other mountain goats in the head, and whichever one ends up with the smallest migraine wins the girl goat.

As for humans? Well, in the old days, it was simple: The caveman with the biggest schlong was thought to be the most fertile, and there you go. With the advent of clothing, it got harder to figure out who was the most hung (at least until the 1970s, when too-tight polyester slacks caused a brief re-surgence of that old tradition). Nowadays, we have different ways of showing our virility—most notably, by the make and model of a man's car. Although, truth be told, I never quite figured that one out; I mean, by that logic it would seem like a woman would pass over the guy driving a stubby little Porsche and head right for the stud piloting his massive Win-nebago around town. Then again, my major was communica-tions, not psychology, so what do I know?

In any case, let's get on back to the wonders of the female anatomy. We've already established that everything is all up inside. But what exactly is this "everything"?

To begin with, there's the vagina. (Yes, I'm going to be talk-ing all "clinical" here. Sorry. You want smut? Go rifle through your dad's nightstand.) This is the first hurdle that your pre-cious sperm must clear before it makes its way to the finish line. Not as easy as it sounds, because, as I hinted at before, it's basically a hostile environment. Enemy territory, if you will.

Remember, the vagina is naturally acidic. This is just an-other of nature's ways of weeding out the good sperm from the bad, figuring, like in New York, if your guys can make it here, they can make it anywhere.

The vagina's acidity is actually a good thing for women, as it helps protect and defend your loved one's nether regions from various bacteria, both foreign and domestic. The bad news, my friend, is that your sperm has been formally classi-fied as an enemy combatant. It's true: Your wife might be saying, "Yes, yes!" but her vagina is saying, "No, no!" while, in effect, waving the jagged neck of a broken beer bottle to-ward you. Oh yeah, this is gonna be fun!

But don't worry, because if you'll remember from earlier, one of the functions of semen is to help neutralize some of that acidity, thus giving your tiny guys a fighting chance.

THE BIG WHITE ONE

Actually, when you think about it, the whole process of insemination is like some really cool superexciting war movie:

A hundred million eager young soldiers are dropped off on an enemy beach by a massive wave of seamen (sorry, but it fits the metaphor). Upon landing, most of them are immediately mowed down by a line of well-dug-in acids and white blood cells. But a small band of hardy few press on and eventually make it past these seemingly impregnable defenses. They are tasked with one mission: Track down and infiltrate their target (her egg) at all costs. Damn, that sounds cool! I can almost hear the theme music now!

As our brave squad of wiggling white commandos penetrates deeper into the dark unknown, they find themselves at the cervix, a tight, muscular piece of tissue that acts as the gateway between the vagina and the uterus, effectively corking up the baby inside as it develops.

After slipping past the cervix, they're into the uterus, the large, pear-shaped organ where (hopefully) the baby itself will be growing. The lining of the uterus, the *endometrium*, is what is shed every month during a woman's period (for more about that, see chapter 3). I'm not going to sugarcoat it: For your sperm, this is their Bataan Death March. You're going to lose a lot more men during this part of the mission—some because they run out of energy, stop swimming, and die, and others because they'll refuse to ask for directions on where to go next. But the strongest and hardiest will soldier on and make it to the final leg of their mission.

Meanwhile, on either side of the uterus are the female equivalent of our testicles: the ovaries. This is where the female sex cell (the oocyte, ova, or egg, depending on how technical you want to get) lives in structures called *follicles*. You'll notice I said "lives," and not "is created," because unlike sperm, which constantly regenerate, women are born with a finite number of follicles. Yes, they're *born with eggs*, one per follicle. In fact, a woman has the highest number of eggs she'll ever have before she's even born—around four million. Unfortunately, it's all downhill from there. Her body is genetically programmed for these follicles to start dying off from the get-go, so the number of egg follicles immediately goes down to one million at birth, and decreases to less than half that when she reaches puberty, with a loss of between five hundred and a thousand eggs per month after that.

Now, once a month, one of her two ovaries releases an egg, sending it down the connecting fallopian tube toward the uterus. Like our sperm, each egg contains a genetic code of twenty-three chromosomes—exactly half a human. It's the job of our plucky squad of sperm, which, incidentally, have now been whittled down to maybe two hundred or so, to intercept that egg, get that code, and, together, make a baby.

They carefully sneak up the fallopian tube, and when they see the egg a-comin' from the other direction, they strike! All the remaining sperm surround the egg and attack, trying to force their way inside. Only one will make it, though, and once he gets in, the egg's defenses activate, shutting out any other competing sperm. Our twenty-three chromosomes mix with her twenty-three chromosomes, and shazam! The egg then finishes its trip down the fallopian tube, where it settles into the uterus (at which point it is considered an *embryo*), and attaches itself to the endometrium, all set to grow into the baby that will one day put a massive dent in your car's left front fender while driving one-handed in front of the Dairy Queen to impress this cute girl who sits next to him in his health class. And the circle of life goes on . . .

Sounds easy, right?

Sure, everything sounds easy in the planning stages. I'm sure it was a piece of cake for someone to say, "Okay, boys, here's the deal. We're going to put some guys in a rocket, shoot them up to the moon, have 'em walk around for a bit, stick a flag in the dirt, maybe hit a couple of golf balls, then we bring them home!" It's the *execution* that can get a bit tricky . . .

I'LL JUST TAKE THE SPERM TO COVER

You like betting on sports? Poring over sheets of stats and calculating the "overs" and "unders" your thing? Great. Then you'll love what I have to tell you next: Even under optimal conditions, the fine art of baby making is a matter of playing the percentages.

According to statistics from the United States Centers for Disease Control, 80 percent of women under the age of thirty-five have a chance of becoming pregnant within the first year they try. In the next two years, 10 percent more will succeed, which leaves the remaining 10 percent, who require some kind of fertility treatment. Unfortunately, of those 10 percent, only *half* of the treatments will succeed, leaving 5 percent of women who will not be able to get pregnant under any circumstances.[b]

Breaking it down by age, thirty-five is usually the landmark when it comes to fertility in women, since it is at this point, generally, that the process of egg degradation kicks into high gear, further limiting the total amount of her "good eggs"—i.e., the ones that have the best chance of being fertilized and developing. This process increases exponentially over the next few years: Two-thirds of women over forty suffer fertility problems, and that number increases to a whopping *95 percent* after the age of forty-six.

This is often seen as patently unfair, biologically speaking, since even though sperm production may diminish as men age, viable sperm can be produced well into a man's eighties and nineties (see: King, Larry or Randall, Tony). If you ask me, this just seems more creepy than unfair; a new father should not need to have *his* diapers changed more frequently than his baby's.

WHA' HAPPEN'D?

So many things can go wrong during fertilization. It's a wonder any babies are born at all: Too few sperm, or too many low-quality sperm, and there won't be enough survivors to make it to the egg; poor ovulation; scarring or cysts in the fallopian tubes that prevent the egg from meeting the sperm; low-quality eggs; the fertilized egg's failure to implant—the list goes on and on.

Infertility can be caused by one or all of these things, as well as a vast number of other genetic issues. But don't lose heart. Your fertility specialist has myriad tests at his disposal (including one involving hamsters—yeah, you heard me, *hamsters*—you'll see) that he can run on both you and your wife to help pinpoint your own particular fertility issues.

Okay, so we're almost there. But, um, there's one more area that we need to cover in the next chapter for you to have a complete overview of the whole reproductive cycle, and how it can be affected by infertility.

The good news is you already know what it is. Well, at least you should. After all, as a married man, you spend twelve long, hard weeks a year dealing with it . . .

THREE

You Need to
Know about This...
Period

*M*enses. The menstrual cycle. Also known as "the Period."

The very mention of the word has been known to cause mighty lumberjacks to break into nervous titters and reduce erudite Ph.D.s to clapping their hands over their ears and yelling, "La la la la la! I can't hear you!"

What women need to know is that they should not take any of these adverse reactions personally. They're merely primal male responses to a completely foreign ability that only women experience—like the capacity to sit through an all-day *Grey's Anatomy* marathon. Personally, in that situation I'd rather gouge out my right eyeball with a shrimp fork, but hey, different strokes . . .

When it comes to our knowledge about the workings of the female sex organs, we men are divided into two groups: the ones who brought the signed parental consent form back in tenth-grade health class and got "the lecture," and those who were sent off to the multipurpose room to watch a PG movie.

Unfortunately, when you're a grown-up and you're in the process of trying to conceive a baby, you don't have the luxury of ignorance. Knowledge of the inner workings of a woman is paramount, and this time no one gets to go and watch *Willy Wonka & the Chocolate Factory* as an "alternate activity."

As a practical analogy, I give you your car. There are plenty of guys who are only interested in what's on the outside—clear-coat paint, spinning rims, flames painted down the sides—and that's all fine. Well, except for the flames. That's actually really lame. If you have those, please get rid of them. No potential father should be driving a giant Hot Wheels car.

With these guys, when something goes wrong with their car, they open up the hood and take a peek, but they have no idea what they're looking at. Oh, sure, every guy likes to brag about what he thinks he knows, but how many of us can actually pop the hood of our ride and tell what's going on? All we see is a tangle of wires and pumps and cables and things with fourteen-digit part numbers written on them in Japanese.

Okay, now try to think of a woman's reproductive system as that car engine—only with a clitoris. Trust me, when you and your partner are entering the wonderful world of fertility treatments, it can only help to know as much as you can about what's going on under her hood—specifically, the ins and outs of the female menstrual cycle. Still with me? Good!

Now roll up those sleeves, throw on some gloves, and get out that little overhead-light-bulb-on-a-hook thing your dad always had hanging on the garage tool wall but never used—and a-here we go!

OH, SHE'S JUST GOING
THROUGH A PHASE

To begin with, what's most commonly called a woman's cycle is actually made up of three separate phases. Now I hear what you're saying: "Oh, you don't have to tell me this stuff! I already know the phases." That's okay. Most men think they do:

- The "Why the heck are you crying? It's just a stupid TV show" phase.

- The "What are you talking about? You're not fat and you have a whole closet full of things to wear!" phase.

- And of course, the "Just-toss-the-family-size-bag-of-Peanut-M&M's-at-her-give-her-the-remote-control-and-back-the-hell-away!" phase.

(IMPORTANT SIDE NOTE: Under *no circumstances* should you share any of these idiotic whack-a-doo theories with your partner, because if you do, you'll quickly enter the "Go sleep at your friend's house, you dumb, insensitive prick!" phase. Best to avoid that phase.)

In real terms, the three phases are commonly known as:

1. The *follicular phase*

2. *Ovulation*

3. The *luteal phase*

Pretty cool medical-sounding stuff, huh? Let me tell you. You learn these names, and you'll be the hit of every cocktail party (as long as you party with gynecologists—if not, try to avoid discussing this topic over drinks).

All of these phases involve the release of hormones—a subject with which, as you embark down the road of fertility treatments, you will become quite intimately involved. Simply put, a hormone is a substance created by the body that has a physiological effect on another part of the body. Okay, in even simpler terms, think of a hormone as that cop who unexpectedly switches lanes and falls in behind you while you're driving. One glance back at that black-and-white cruiser in your rearview mirror and all of a sudden you're a law-abiding, precise, and courteous driver. And that's what a hormone does—it effects change.

So, want to find out what happens during the period? Well, too bad, because we're going to look at it anyway.

A MENSTRUAL CYCLE BUILT FOR TWO

To begin with, there is a difference between what's commonly called a menstrual "period" and a menstrual "cycle." A period denotes the amount of time it takes for a woman to shed the inner lining of her uterus (the actual menstruation, or "bleeding"), which usually lasts through days one through five of a woman's menstrual cycle. The reason this lining builds up in the first place is to support the implantation of a possible baby (think back to your bachelor days, when you'd only clean up your apartment and make it look nice if you knew someone was coming over later). If her body doesn't sense an embryo implanting, it doesn't need the lining, and out it comes.

If you're like most guys, right now you're cringing and have that look on your face reserved for those people in cop shows who are called to the morgue to identify a body and the detective pulls back the sheet saying something like, "Yeah, the rats pretty much ate half of his face, but is this your friend?" You know; it's weird. We can watch movies like *300* and *Saving Private Ryan* all day long, with guys hacking off arms and legs while carrying their own intestines—but a little vaginal bleeding and boom! We're on the floor.

On a personal note, Julie and I have worked out a carefully constructed agreement to alleviate any potentially awkward moments in this area: When it's her time of the month, after she takes care of all her "female business" in the bathroom, she discreetly throws away any applicators or wrappers, carefully and methodically making sure all evidence of the act is completely disposed of. This way, there is no danger of me running out of the bathroom screaming like a little girl if I find a used tampon floating in the toilet. It's a simple system, but it works!

In contrast to the period, a menstrual cycle lasts anywhere from twenty-five to thirty-one days, and includes all of the phases mentioned above. It is important for both you and your partner to know the difference, as most fertility methods involve keeping careful track of the phases in order to predict the optimum time for conception. Some women have longer cycles than others, so don't automatically assume that it's exactly thirty days.

A cycle is like a revolving credit card account: With some cards the payment is due on the first of the month, and with others it may be the third. Or the fifth. And then there are those cards that offer you a sports team logo of your choice and special 0 percent financing that somehow magically disappears after six months, and then they go and jack up the interest rate to 30 percent and your minimum payment doubles and now you're broke and all you have to show for it is a MasterCard with some cheesy little 49ers helmet on it and a 380 credit score! But I digress . . .

Long story short: To keep your finances in order, you need to know when your credit card payment due date is so you can be sure to make your payments on time. Similarly, for successful fertility methods, you need to know when your partner's cycle begins, when she ovulates, and when she gets her period so you can keep track of when to put in your, um . . . *payments.*

Now I hear you saying, "Okay, Greg—I think I understand the difference between a period and a menstrual cycle, and I definitely get that you're not a fan of a cashless economy. But why is it important for me to know how long her cycle is? What difference does it make, anyway?" Tell you what—let's flag that question for right now, because before we go any further with how all of this relates to infertility, you'll need to learn the timeline for your partner's cycle, and how it breaks down.

FOLLICULAR? I BARELY KNOW HER!

To recap, days one through five of a woman's cycle are what is commonly referred to as her *period*, or *menstruation*—the shedding of the unused endometrium (the lining of the uterus).

While this is happening, surges of hormones (remember them?) are simultaneously being released from the pituitary gland in the brain and from inside the ovaries, which trigger several of the many egg follicles inside the ovaries to begin to grow. Then, usually on day six, the *follicular phase* begins

As I mentioned before, a woman is born with around one million immature eggs in her ovaries, a staggering number, but because of natural forces in her body, that dwindles down to around 400,000 to 450,000 by puberty—which is still a pretty respectable amount. Now before you start imagining the horrors of a half-million diaper changes a day, or even worse, begin contemplating the creation of your own private clone army sequestered in a remote volcano hideout like some megalomaniacal villain bent on world conquest, you should know that a normal ovary releases only one, maybe two eggs during ovulation, and her hormones will cause about one thousand more to self-destruct per month. Sorry, dude—the world will have to wait. Besides, do you know what the upkeep is on a volcano hideout?

During the follicular phase, one dominant egg emerges from those few stimulated follicles, which then triggers the lining of the uterus to start to thicken and ready itself for a possible implantation. It usually takes ten to fourteen days to mature an egg, so by now we're in the middle of the whole cycle. This is when things really get moving. *Literally.*

IT'S NOT OVER TILL IT'S OVA

At this phase in the cycle, called *ovulation*, the lucky egg (or ova) breaks free from its follicle and begins to travel down the fallopian tube toward the uterus, which is still preparing itself for its potential visitor. If there's any sperm in the woman's reproductive system, this is when and where the two of them will hook up, but it's not as easy as it sounds. Remember, for the last few days your sperm have been swimming all the way up through the cervix and down the fallopian tubes, so it's going to be a bit tired if and when it does meet up with the egg.

By comparison, think of having to run two or three Ironman triathlons, and right as you finish the last leg you're taken to a conference room where you're then expected to give a perfect presentation to a client that will make or break your career. Maybe a *little* bit of pressure?

This is also the time during which your partner may experience a bit of pain in her abdomen or pelvic area, called *mittelschmerz* (German for "middle pain," which makes pretty good sense, since it's a pain in her middle—you can't accuse the Germans of mincing words, can you?). It can be caused by follicular swelling, her fallopian tubes contracting, irritation because of fluid buildup—none of which are serious conditions, mind you—and generally lasts up to a few hours.

(IMPORTANT NOTE: This is a *minor* pain, and should be treated as such. You'll have plenty of time to dote on her hand and foot later on during the fertility treatments and when she's pregnant. On the scale of errands you're obligated to run for her—a sliding scale in which your tasks become more and more elaborate the more discomfort your wife is in—this one rates a "go out and get her some ice cream, but only if you feel like you want some too.")

GET OVER HERE AND PLANT ONE IN ME

Meanwhile, the follicle that released the egg has a job to do as well. The remnants of the follicle will transform into something called the *corpus luteum*—which means that we are now in the aptly named *luteal phase*. See how all of this is starting to make some kind of crazy sense? (Even if it doesn't, just smile and nod your head, then reread the chapter. I promise you'll get it. Your mother and I have a lot of faith in you.)

It's the vital job of this corpus luteum to release *progesterone* and *estrogen*, two key hormones that help stabilize the endometrium and prepare it for the arrival (and, hopefully, the implantation) of the fertilized egg. It's kind of like making a reservation at the uterus: "Oh, and if you can make it a spot near the cervix, that'd be great!"

As a side note, you'll do well to remember the words "progesterone" and "estrogen." They're the peanut butter and jelly of most fertility treatments. More about them later. Lots more.

Normally, a woman's temperature will rise by a degree or two during this luteal phase, which is why you'll find so many couples on constant thermometer watch to help tell them when is the best time to try to conceive. Strike while the iron's hot, so to speak. Unfortunately, this is inexact science at best. "But why?" you ask. Whoa, there! Slow it down a second. I mean, up until a couple of paragraphs ago you didn't even know what a corpus luteum was, and now you're getting all worked up? Relax—we'll be taking a look at this special relationship between woman, menstrual cycle, and thermometer in just a bit. First, let's consider timing . . .

NEAT TRIVIA THAT PROBABLY WON'T IMPRESS YOUR POKER BUDDIES IN THE LEAST . . .

The exact time your partner ovulates really depends on the *true length* of her cycle. (See? I told you they wouldn't be impressed. Okay, you can also tell them that Christopher Walken was originally considered for the role of Han Solo in *Star Wars*. That should shut them up.)

Many women trying to get pregnant believe that since normal ovulation is supposed to occur on day fourteen, they should have sex on days twelve, thirteen, or fourteen, because sperm can stay in the system for up to four days. Makes sense. After all, you want that sperm all ready and waiting with candy and flowers to meet that little egg as it starts coming down the pipe, right? Well, maybe not.

Many women ovulate earlier or later than day fourteen—and that's why we need to know exactly on which day of her cycle she ovulates, in order to figure out the right time to "do the deed." Because if you don't, all those sperm you threw in there on day fourteen (thinking that's the right day) might not have an egg to fertilize. And since they're male sperm, you know they won't even try to ask anyone for directions, so they'll just keep swimming around until they die. How typical. So let's take a look at a few different ways she can get the timing right.

I'M HAVING A CHART ATTACK!

You wake up in the morning. You had a great night of sleep, and you're ready for the day. You roll over to kiss your wife good morning—and nearly get your eye impaled by the thermometer sticking out of her mouth. Don't worry, though, she's not sick. She's *charting*, which is basically trying to learn, on average over the course of a few months, on which day her ovulation takes place.

Luckily, this is the part of fertility that you barely have to worry about. Yep, just like how your wife is in control of your social calendar and she tells you that you're having dinner with the Pattersons next Saturday—even though you completely hate them because they spend the whole meal raving about some weird foreign art film they saw. But when you say you just saw a cool action flick they look at you like you're something they found clinging to the fur under their cat's tail. Anyway, she's in charge of charting her fertility cycle.

However, since I'm trying to be thorough, and because I know how much my wife used to light up when it looked like I was actually interested in knowing what she was doing during this time (and we all know how important it is to score those "relationship points" when we can), I'll take you through a quick tour of what your partner is up to.

Like I said earlier, she knows all the ins and outs of this, but what it basically comes down to is keeping track of different aspects of her body in order to predict when the best time would be for her to get pregnant. This can be accomplished a few ways:

1. **Temperature:** She keeps track of what is called her "basal body temperature" (BBT) by taking her temperature every morning. Remember when I said that after she ovulates, all of those delightful little hormones go rushing through her body? Well, not only do those hormones, namely progesterone, make her an absolute delight to be around, but they also raise her body temperature anywhere from 0.4° to 0.8° in order to get her insides in the best possible shape for her (hopefully) fertilized egg.

   Here's a little known fact: You know how in all of those movies and TV shows you see a woman taking her temperature, looking at the thermometer, and then screaming to her husband, "Okay! My temperature is up! Let's do it!" and then she jumps on him and they have this incredibly spontaneous, fun, and awesome sex, and the baby is conceived? Yeah, that's pretty much a load of crap.

   The reality is that by the time her temperature goes up, it's already too late. The proverbial egg ship has sailed, and Mr. Sperm is left waiting on the dock, tail-deep in all that confetti. (What, you never watched *The Love Boat*?)

So what good does all this temperature taking do? Well, it helps give her a better idea of when she *did* ovulate that month, which in turn helps her plan out when her peak fertility time might be for the following month—and *that's* when she yells, "It's time!" and jumps on you. While all this planning can definitely be a big help with conception, the pressure of having to get it on at a precise time month after month makes sex . . . well, about as exciting as doing the laundry. (Actually, the laundry might be slightly more exciting, depending on how many different types of clothes you tend to wash and at what temperatures.)

Never fear though, as later on we'll discuss some ways to make the "baby-making sex" a lot more exciting! Well, somewhat more exciting. Okay, *tolerable*.

2. **Cervical mucus method:** This one has to do with the changes that will be happening in regard to her vaginal chemistry. In the days leading up to ovulation, your wife's cervix will begin to produce a mucus, which is intended to make it easier for sperm to make its way through. The closer it gets to her ovulation, the thicker and more viscous the mucus will become, oftentimes compared to, um, raw egg whites, and . . . you know what? You're better off letting her handle this one.

3. **Ovulation prediction:** The gold standard. These ovulation tests that she can buy in any market or drugstore look exactly like those little pee sticks that tell her if she's pregnant or not, except these are designed specifically to tell her when she is about to ovulate. Without getting too technical (but still giving you enough info to impress your significant other), the test measures for surges of *luteinizing hormone* (LH)—the hormone released by the pituitary gland that triggers ovulation.

Now I hear what you're saying, "Luteinizing hormone? But that sounds like it would have something to do with the 'luteal phase.' And doesn't that come *after* ovulation? Sorry, Greg, I just don't get it." You know what? That's perfectly fine.

See, I have this theory that the whole menstrual process was designed to be so confusing and impenetrable to the male mind that it would naturally drive men away from digging too deep—because if we did, we would uncover a secret so terrible, so impossibly horrific, that it would shatter our minds beyond repair and tear our souls asunder.

So in my humble opinion, to avoid bringing about any possible apocalypse, it's better just to shut up and let her pee on the stick. She knows what she's doing, even if you don't.

Now don't get too concerned if it seems like she's peeing on them all the time at first. It's kind of like when we guys get ourselves a new piece of stereo equipment. You know, except we kind of skip that "peeing on it" part. Or maybe you don't. I don't know; nor do I judge.

WHERE DOES SHE GET THOSE WONDERFUL TOYS?

In addition to these methods, there is a whole cottage industry of other handy little gadgets out there that can help you along with the charting, as well as dozens of fertility Web sites with automatic calendars that she can plug all her numbers and dates into, and then, when it's time, she'll get a message that says, well, "It's time." Your wife is undoubtedly fully versed on all of these, and I'm sure she will be more than happy to spend hours upon hours explaining all of these wonders to you if you give her a chance. The trick is don't give her that chance.

Once again—and I can't stress this enough—these charting activities should be looked upon as your wife's domain. You wouldn't want her second-guessing you as you pick out the right drill bit to put up shelves in the den, would you?

Plus, and I'm saying this with all due love and respect, she may not have the patience to explain such delicate scientific machinations to a big dumb ape like you. So here's a simple solution: Give her a hug and kiss, and then say (with that oh-so-charming big-dumb-ape smile of yours), "Wow, that's great honey! So, why don't I just leave you to this, and you can let me know when we have to 'do it.' Okay?" If all goes well, she'll flip her hair that way that you love, smile back, and say, "Okay." And everything should be okay. Okay?

WE PREFER THE TERM "LUTEALLY CHALLENGED," THANK YOU!

If things still don't seem to be tracking right, you can also ask your doctor to run some blood tests to see if your partner's hormone levels are where they should be. If not, they can be tweaked up or down to help regulate her cycles.

In the case of my wife, Julie, and me, it was good that she went in for those tests, since we were able to find out that her luteal phase was too short, a common problem among infertile couples. What happens is that the luteal hormones, the ones a woman needs to make her uterus "nice and fluffy," as my wife's gynecologist so descriptively put it, aren't released for a long enough time, and thus aren't really getting a chance to work. With a shortened luteal phase, even if an egg is lucky enough to be fertilized, it would have no place to implant. In other words, it throws *everything* off.

Fortunately, in the case of my wife, it was just a matter of finding the right hormone cocktail and, just like that, problem solved. (Well, *her* problem was solved. As it turned out, I had some reproductive issues of my own to deal with, but since I don't have a uterus, let's save that one for later, shall we?)

So there we are—now you know the basics of your partner's fertility cycle, and are ready to continue your quest for fertility knowledge, confident in the fact that you can tell a cycle from a period, and a corpus luteum from mittel-schmerz. Do me a favor though. Please don't go and buy that lame AMATEUR GYNECOLOGIST T-shirt that they sell at tourist shops at the beach. Not cool.

FOUR

Let's All Play the
Blame Game!

*D*octors technically define infertility as a couple's inability to achieve a pregnancy after one year of trying. During that year, as time ticks by and nothing seems to be happening, a lot of questions run through your mind. As a man, the chief of which is: Whose fault is this?

As a guy, we have a natural tendency to try to fix things. How many times has your wife complained about something at home, at work, or in her personal life, and you offer some kind of fix, and what do you get for your aid? You get *yelled at*! "I didn't need an answer!"

Of course, we have no idea what the hell just happened, since when we're with our buddies, and one of them shares a problem, he's obviously looking for advice and/or help. After all, who complains just to complain?

Your wife, that's who.

As a guy, when you see a hole in the wall, sure you want to fix it, but the first thing you want to know is, "How did that happen? Who did it?" Unfortunately, too often when a very sensitive situation like infertility comes up, we bring what I like to call "man-logic" to the problem. We want to know *why* this is happening, why it's happening to us, and whose fault it is. After all, when the Steelers lose, we don't just say, "That's too bad. Maybe next time." We say, "Son of a bitch! We would have won if the ref hadn't blown that call! And yeah, if we'd scored twenty-one more points that would've helped too." We need someone or something to blame. It's not good or bad. It's just . . . us.

In our minds, we're all virile testosterone-fueled baby-making machines. Hell, the only reason we don't already have a trail of babies all over the country is because we were *really* careful back in our twenties. And so, using this man-logic, if there's any fault to be had, it is placed firmly upon the shoulders of our significant others. After all, there's so much going on inside her that whatever's wrong *must* be her problem. So all she needs to do is relax and let things take their course and it'll be fine.

Yeah, tell her that. I dare you.

FIX THE PROBLEM, NOT THE BLAME

According to the American Society for Reproductive Medicine, the reasons for infertility are pretty much split up evenly between the sexes with male problems as the cause somewhere around a third of the time, female problems another third, and a his/hers combo plate of around 10 percent. For the remaining 20–25 percent of infertility cases, the causes are completely . . . unexplained (cue the eerie music).[c]

But, just for your own peace of mind, let's look at some of the possible reasons you two just aren't getting the job done:

BLUE GENES

Genetics can play a large role in not being able to conceive. There are several genetic disorders that can prevent fertilization, some of which you've heard of, like cystic fibrosis, and some of which you haven't, like Klinefelter's or Turner syndromes. There may even be issues with your chromosomes themselves, which, if you'll recall, are the genetic blueprints that come half from the father, half from the mother.

Not all genetic disorders necessarily present themselves outwardly, so just because you aren't sporting a hunchback and spitting acid, don't think you're automatically in the clear. You still need to be tested to see if any of these genetic abnormalities may possibly be hampering your fertility. At this point, medical science is so advanced that they can take a blood sample from you and determine exactly *which gene* on *which chromosome* may be abnormal. Think about how cool and amazing that is for a second. I mean this is real *Star Trek*-level stuff. But no, they can't go in and rewrite your DNA to make you superstrong while they're at it. That's a stupid question. Besides, I already asked.

Now if it turns out that your problem isn't genetic, that's good. At this point the doctor can move on to take a look at more of the physical, mechanical problems that may be holding you two back from potential dirty-diaper duty. Obviously, as each sex is different, each has its own problems to deal with, and since this is a book for and about men, what say we start with you?

THERE'S A PROBLEM
WITH MY MALE DELIVERY

As the old saying goes, I've got good news and I've got bad news. The good news is that there's usually only one problem when it comes to male infertility. The bad news is that that problem concerns pretty much the *only* thing that you bring to the fertilization party—your sperm.

To make a baby, your sperm needs to swim long and far enough to reach, and penetrate, the egg. That's it. End of story. If it doesn't or isn't able to—for any reason—that is considered a male fertility problem. Yeah, there can be a lot of reasons why your sperm may not be up to snuff, such as low numbers, poor shape, or lack of swimming ability (see chapter 7, Sperm-A-Lot, for more details), but the bottom line is, well, that's the bottom line.

First of all, you're going to have to hand over a sample. The doctor can get it from you in one of two ways: One you know very well and the other . . .

The first is obviously masturbation into a collection cup. Chapter 7 goes into some of the protocols and particulars of that little trip to the doctor's office. The second way is a bit more . . . involved. Its technical name is *microscopic epididymal sperm aspiration* (MESA for short). It's a procedure in which sperm cells are extracted directly from your *epididymis* (a tiny tube in your scrotum that is basically the train station for your sperm cells where they wait to catch the "Semen Express"), and it involves, well, needles. Yeah. Think of it as the difference between your sperm agreeing to surrender and come out quietly with their tails up, and having the SWAT team bust the door down to go in and get 'em.

Now if you're really running dry, or if your plumbing is clogged beyond all repair, the technique of last resort is *testicular sperm extraction* (a.k.a. TESE), where a small piece of your . . . um, testicle, is removed, and what few sperm cells might be hanging around in there are extracted, tested, and then used to fertilize an egg. You do this, and you're a hero. Seriously. Yeah, it's done under anesthesia, but even the thought of this procedure can cause guys to pass out, so if you're one of those unlucky few, my hat's off to you.

There are a wide variety of tests your fertility doctor can, and will, run on your semen to get to the root cause of what's going on. Make no mistake. Your little guys are gonna be put through the ringer, with a series of trials and exercises that make Navy SEAL training look like a jog on the beach.

Some of the basic tests will examine your semen for:

- **Sperm endurance:** They leave your sperm out in a dish for three hours, and then come back and see how many are still alive. The number should be around 50 percent.

- **Semen thickness:** Basically, if you find yourself ejaculating something with the consistency of fresh Vermont maple syrup, not enough sperm may be able to pull free from the goop to start swimming toward the cervix.

- **Fructose:** Yeah, as in the sugar. If there's too much of it in your semen, it could be the sign of a blocked *seminal vesicle* (one of a pair of glands sitting behind your bladder that produce more than half of your seminal fluid). Of course, you could just have a completely messed-up method of drinking orange juice. Either way, it's not a good thing.

Now depending on what these tests show, and if the doctor suspects there may be some kind of blockage happening up in there, he may decide you need even more detailed testing. And that's when he has to pull out the big guns. Now, though some of these tests have a very definite "mad scientist" vibe going on, don't worry, they do the job.

- **Vasography:** The doctor will make a small incision in your scrotum, then inject some dye into your testicles, and x-ray the whole thing to try to find the blockage. You can stop squeezing your legs together now. The procedure is done under general anesthesia. You won't feel a thing. Promise.

- **Transrectal ultrasound:** A probe is inserted into—gee, guess where?—and used to check for blockages in the seminal vesicles. This is probably the test you're most likely to skip when you're recounting the whole deal to your buddies.

- **Testicular biopsy:** Okay, for this one you can squeeze your legs together again. The doctor takes a small sample from your testicle to see if there's any healthy sperm swimming around in there. If so, you probably have a blockage.

- **Hamster-sperm penetration test:** Your sperm is mixed with hamster eggs to see how many can actually penetrate. That's it. You really need me to make a joke for this one?

In the interest of full disclosure, yes, some of these tests can be . . . uncomfortable. But remember: You're a man and your wife is counting on you to do your part in this. If it helps, you can pretend you've been shot down behind enemy lines and you're being interrogated. Just grit your teeth, grab the exam table, and only give 'em your name, rank, and medical insurance group number.

So by now you've been poked and prodded so much that you might feel like a UFO abductee. Generally, if you happen to be the one with the problem, by this time the doctor will likely be able to identify it—and you'll have some war stories to last the rest of your life.

OKAY, LET'S PUT 'ER UP ON THE RACK AND SEE WHAT WE GOT

Now, let's take a look at your wife. As you've learned, she's got a lot more moving parts in there. What with her hormones and fallopian tubes and endometrial lining and whatnot. In a nutshell, you are a set of pipes, while she, on the other hand, is a fine Swiss timepiece.

In truth, the analogy isn't that far off: Her complex reproductive system has to run like clockwork in order for her egg to be released at just the right time, meet your sperm to be fertilized, and then travel down to embed itself in the uterus.

Okay, quick review: In chapter 3, you learned all about her menstrual cycle. Remember all that stuff about the follicular and luteal phases, how they release her eggs, and so on and so forth? Good, then here's a tougher one: Do you remember what *triggers* these phases? Yep, hormones. Hormones are the keys to making sure everything runs exactly the way it's supposed to, and she's got a lot of them swirling around in there.

Say you go out for a night of drinking with the boys. (Yes, I know, as you're a married guy this scenario exists in a fanciful world populated by dragons, unicorns, and *Star Wars* prequels that didn't crap all over your fond adolescent memories, but work with me here.) You walk up to the bar and decide to order a martini—vodka, vermouth, maybe some olive juice (and, obviously, shaken not stirred). Now, if the bartender throws in too much vermouth, the drink ends up too dry. Too much vodka, it's got too much bite. Too much olive juice, and it becomes liquid *tapas*. No, in order to make a perfect martini, your barman will have to carefully mix exactly the correct amounts of liquors in just the right order. Take a minute and think about the delicate intricacies of the beverage next time you order one up—then go ahead and get yourself nice and plowed.

Now this same basic idea of perfect mixology can be applied to your wife and that crazy concoction of hormones she's got sloshing around inside of her. Too much of one hormone is just as bad as too little of another, and either one could cause her whole menstrual cycle to—well, I believe the technical term would be "go all whack-a-doo." Needless to say, this is a bad thing—for everyone involved.

So, the first thing your doctor is going to check is her hormone levels, to make sure things are happening at the right time for the right *amount* of time. These tests can also tell how many eggs she still has in her reserves, based on the amount of hormones it takes to prime an egg for release during her ovulation. The higher certain hormone levels read, the more it's taking to prep her eggs, which could signal low reserves of "good eggs."

When you look at this in the context of man's continuing quest for scientific knowledge, and how much we've advanced in our understanding of the human body, it's absolutely mind-boggling that within only the last few years doctors have been able to decode and interpret these complex hormonal signals and what they mean in terms of a woman's fertility—and yet to this day I still can't drive under a freeway overpass without my AM radio going all static-y on me. Weird.

In any case, your doctor will be able to better explain the actual levels involved, and how they may be affecting your partner's fertility, as it can vary greatly from woman to woman.

POLYCYSTIC OVARIES? HEY,
MY COUSIN GRADUATED FROM THERE!

The most common hormonal problem you may encounter is *polycystic ovarian syndrome*, which is literally translated as "ovaries containing many cysts." It affects somewhere around 10 percent of all women, and is serious enough to be a definite cause of fertility problems.

About half of women with polycystic ovarian syndrome (PCOS) are overweight, and although the final verdict's still pending on which comes first, the syndrome or the weight gain, many doctors believe the hormone imbalance that causes PCOS is what causes the weight gain, and not vice versa. This makes things twice as hard, as studies have shown that weight gain tends to decrease the chances of pregnancy.

Now this part gets complicated, so pay attention: With PCOS, something in the body tells it to start making too much insulin, which is the hormone that helps regulate blood sugar. When insulin production goes into overdrive, two things happen within the woman: 1) weight gain, and 2) increase in male hormone production. Yes, *male hormones*.

So what happens then? Well, the woman begins to exhibit a number of biological phenomena we most commonly associate with being "male": thinning hair or baldness, excess facial hair, acne, and forgetting to take out the trash cans on Thursday night for Friday morning pickup.

These male hormones get in the way of her female hormones, and screw up what they're supposed to be doing. Inside her ovaries, the eggs produced in her egg follicle will rise to the top like normal, but they won't release. This causes the follicle to fill with fluid continuously until it swells up, creating something called a *follicular cyst*. These eventually burst, and the egg is lost. Yikes. The cysts themselves can cause some pain, but really, that's not the dangerous part.

The problem arises when these cysts become chronic. See, if no eggs are ever released, then there's never going to be any ovulation. Without ovulation, there can be no menstruation. And without menstruation, the lining of the uterus isn't shed, which can lead to thick tissue buildup, which can then lead to cancer. Needless to say, this is an issue that needs to be diagnosed and treated as early as possible.

THIS UTERUS HAS BEEN RED TAGGED

In addition to the potential hormone problems, there is also the possibility of structural problems within the female reproductive system. An analogy can be made to moving into a new home.

If you buy a new home, but the building itself isn't architecturally sound, you can't live inside. Furthermore, if the bridge leading to the building has been closed, and you can't get the U-Haul full of your stuff to its destination, that's another reason you're not going to be moving in any time soon. The same holds true for the uterus and its surrounding organs. There are several possible issues with the uterus and/or fallopian tubes that can hamper fertility:

- **Fibroids:** Sporting a name that conjures the image of a latex-masked alien in an old *Doctor Who* episode, fibroids are benign tumors found inside or outside the uterus. When inside the uterus, they may grow to crowd the walls and not permit an egg to implant, or they may make the space too small for a fetus to grow at all. These can be surgically removed, the severity of the surgery depending on the size and placement of the fibroids.

- **Polyps:** These are small growths inside the uterus. They are usually not a major problem, but too many can interfere with implantation. These, too, are usually removed with a simple surgery.

Either of these issues can potentially make the uterus architecturally unsound—and unsafe for potential occupants. But before you hang a CONDEMNED sign around your wife's waist, relax. In many of these cases, your doctor can help bring your wife up to code.

ENDOMETRIOSIS

I'm giving this problem its own section (and without a funny title), not only because this is such a strange one, but also because it's an extremely common issue in the world of infertility. According to the Endometriosis Research Center, around 10 million American women are afflicted by it and it is the cause of over *35 percent* of all infertility issues.[d]

"Okay, enough of the dramatic buildup," you say. "What is it?" Well, it's basically the growth of endometrial tissue (which, you'll remember, is the lining of the uterus) in other places in the body. Now when I say "other places in the body" I'm not talking about only those places in and around the other reproductive organs surrounding the uterus, such as the ovaries and fallopian tubes, but also those places you'd never expect to see it—like the liver, kidneys, lungs, skin, and even the brain. The theory is that some wayward endometrial cells set out for greener pastures and somehow travel through the circulatory system, implanting wherever they happen to end up, whether they're welcome there or not— sort of a biological Manifest Destiny. (Sorry, that's the social studies teacher in me coming out. But if you don't know what that is, shame on you.)

Now here comes the really gross part: Because it's endometrial tissue, when a woman's hormones signal that it is time for her period, this tissue starts to bleed—wherever it might be located in the body. Normally, when the endometrial tissue in the uterus bleeds, it has somewhere to go. As in *out*. Not so much when it's in the fallopian tubes or the lungs. So what happens? The surrounding tissues become engorged with blood, inflamed, and eventually injured, resulting in pain, scarring, and all-around badness.

If this scarring occurs in or around the fallopian tubes, it can potentially stop them from picking up and transporting the egg from the ovaries to the uterus—and there you have your "closed bridge."

Can it be treated? Depends. If it's minor scarring or lesions, then yes, they can be removed, one at a time. In the event of major scarring or blockages, though, fertility treatments that bypass the fallopian tubes, such as IVF, may be your only choice. Again, you want to make sure you talk with your doctor about all of the available options.

BUT WAIT . . . THERE'S MORE (MAYBE)

In addition to testing for any or all of the above issues, there are several secondary tests your doctor may want to give your wife in order to identify all possible causes of fertility problems and to be able to prescribe the best course of action.

Along the way, you as a man will discover an interesting fact: While most all of these tests involve checking for various blockages in the ovaries and/or fallopian tubes, or sampling hormone levels at various times during her ovulation cycle for any irregularities, not one of them involves the insertion of rectal probes or the utilization of small rodents (see: hamster-sperm test) like the secondary tests for men.

To me, this provides overwhelming evidence of two things: 1) that men and women have vastly different, though equally important, roles in the reproductive cycle, and 2) that fertility doctors are purposely out to completely screw with us guys every single step of the way.

Okay, maybe not so much number two, but wow, sometimes it can sure feel like it, huh?

FIVE

Great. Now
What the Hell
Are We
Supposed to Do?

*N*eedless to say, it's a huge emotional blow to find out that having the kid you've always wanted isn't going to be a piece of cake. For that matter, it's not even going to be a slice of pie, a sliver of cobbler, or any serving size of your favorite dessert. No, this adds a whole new dimension to the breeding process.

So here we are: The doctor has told you that either you, your wife, or both of you are having fertility problems, and that a "natural" pregnancy is probably out of the question. No matter what the root cause may have turned out to be, whether genetic or medical, you're still going to be faced with that immense question all couples in your situation must confront: "Now what?"

CAN'T I JUST, YOU KNOW, PICK A NUMBER OR SOMETHING?

When it became increasingly clear that Julie and I were going to have to try at least some kind of fertility treatment, quite frankly we were stunned. We both seemed young and healthy. Fertility treatments are what those parents of octuplets do. All we wanted was one lousy kid. Well, one *good* kid, but at that point we would have settled for lousy.

So now we needed to figure out what the game plan was going to be. We knew it was my sperm that was less than quality, which made our decision a bit easier since we didn't have to worry about a lack of eggs. But still, it's not as easy as say, ordering up a fast-food value meal (i.e., there is no "number four in vitro combo"). Each protocol is custom ordered to your particular situation.

Now you and your wife need to have a discussion as to what to do next, and you have a lot of options. But certain options are more appropriate for a given situation than others. Perhaps another "guy metaphor" might be in order . . .

"OH, BEAUTIFUL CHIP SHOT. . . RIGHT UP INTO THE CERVIX!"

Think of infertility as a golf course. A real bitch of a golf course—something Arnold Palmer would have cooked up one Sunday morning while nursing a wicked hangover, and every single hole looks more difficult than the last. Some have sand traps. Some have water hazards. Some have the pin so freakin' far away that all you can do is haul off and swing as hard as you can and hope you land *somewhere* near the green. A wave of helplessness overwhelms you, and you decide to bail on the whole thing and go home and alphabetize your medicine cabinet instead.

But fear not, because confidently striding out from the clubhouse is the course pro (your fertility doctor, for our purposes). Now over the years he's seen lots of guys try to play this course, and he has a pretty good idea of what clubs to use and when (read: what fertility techniques might work the best in your given situation). If you pay attention to what he has to say—and maybe buy him a lemonade around the ninth hole—you might just be able to get out of there under par and set the course record (which would be . . . well, I guess it would be your baby; hey, I never said *every* golfing metaphor was going to be gold).

There are a lot of different protocols your doctor may choose from, and some may be a combination of several strung together, all of which fall under the banner of what is commonly known as ART (*assisted reproduction technology*). So in the interest of you holding up your end and at least appearing to know some of the things your wife is telling you, let's take a look at some of the most common ART protocols, beginning with the easiest, relatively speaking.

CLOMID—C'MON, ISN'T THE NAME FUNNY ENOUGH?

If it's a better, stronger egg you're looking for, then brother, does science have a drug for you. Its technical name is clomiphene citrate, but you can just call it Clomid. It's cool like that. Usually administered as a five-day pill regimen, Clomid is prescribed when all of the equipment in both partners has checked out A-OK (no blockages or medical problems), but the doctor still feels that a little *nudge* to the ovaries might be needed to get things moving—fertility jumper cables, if you will.

Even though some may regard this as the most "basic" fertility drug (if you can call a fertility drug basic), the way Clomid actually works is really interesting, if not downright sneaky:

You know how back when you were single, there always seemed to be that one guy who, even though he was a monster jerk, always had women falling all over him? You know the type: He treats women badly, ignores them, always makes them feel like they aren't thin enough or good-looking enough or whatever, but instead of walking away from him, the girls end up doing anything they can just to try and make him happy. Well, basically, that's how Clomid acts. It's the asshole of the fertility drug world.

See, what happens is once Clomid's been introduced into a woman's body, it slides right up next to her hypothalamus (the organ in the brain that controls hormone production), looks it up and down, smiles, and says, "Yeah, you're not bad looking, but..."

Thrown off-balance, the sweet, innocent young hypothalamus nervously asks, "But...? But what?"

Clomid sighs as it coolly flicks its cigarette to the ground. "Well," it drawls (yeah, in my mind Clomid has a drawl—deal with it), "the thing is, I just don't think you're producing enough estrogen for my taste. But hey, baby, whatever you want to do..."

"No! Wait! I can change—really! Watch!" So the poor little hypothalamus gets herself all in a tizzy and sends a signal to the body to pump out more estrogen, whether it needs to or not. This increased estrogen level causes a hormonal chain reaction that ends with massive amounts of FSH (*follicle stimulating hormone*, which tells the ovaries it's time to grow an immature follicle) and LH (luteinizing hormone, which, as we found out before, actually triggers the ovulation process) being released into her body. The result is that a normal ovary is exposed to a whole lotta the body's own hormones so that bigger, stronger eggs are formed—and in some cases, more than one egg at a time. This is why there is an increased frequency of twins born to couples who use Clomid.

Clomid also has the ability to improve the odds for the eggs it helps to trigger, in that it causes the corpus luteum to produce more progesterone. Remember, the higher the progesterone level, the stickier the endometrium of the uterus gets, and the better chance the egg has of implanting (see chapter 3).

But, like everything, there are the inevitable downsides. In this case, the greatest one would be the risk of multiple pregnancies due to stimulation of more than one egg follicle at a time. Most of the cases of multiple births (triplets, quads, quints, etc.) are due to fertility drugs like Clomid; all of which is fine if you're looking to star in your own reality show, but kind of a drag if you weren't looking to raise what amounts to a baseball team.

The other caveat is that because Clomid tricks your wife's body into thinking it's light on estrogen, her body may react in the same way it would as if she were going through menopause. Your doctor can easily fix this with a little extra estrogen, so definitely let him know if your wife exhibits any possible menopause-like side effects, such as headaches, hot flashes, blurred vision, or keeping a crystal bowl full of butterscotch hard candies on the living room table.

AI . . . AI . . . ? OH . . .

Artificial insemination. Ah, the sound of it is so . . . well, I want to say "romantic," but all that seems to come out is "sci-fi" and/or "creepy." Oddly enough, it does sound a whole lot better than its other name: *intrauterine insemination* (IUI). But, if I may paraphrase Shakespeare, "A fertility protocol by any other name . . ." Whatever you want to call it, it's basically taking your sperm and putting it inside of her vagina, minus the nice dinner and candles.

As with Clomid, this method is best suited for couples who have few to no problems with things like blockages or low sperm counts. In order to get the best result, IUI is often used in conjunction with a follicular stimulant, such as Clomid, to make sure there's at least one or two good eggs for your sperm to hook up with. Without that extra stimulation, there's really no statistical difference between using IUI and just trying to time things right and going for it the old-fashioned way (see chapter 3)—well, other than the fact that with the latter you may have to pop for that dinner/candles scenario after all.

So, what exactly happens with IUI that's so different from timed intercourse? Think of it as your sperm being escorted past the velvet rope directly into Club Uterus—and given an all-access pass to the VIP section to boot. And since the sperm is being introduced directly via catheter, it doesn't have to make that whole long exhausting swim, which means more sperm survive and thus have more chances to hit the egg (or eggs, since Clomid is being used).

Plus, this particular batch of sperm is going to the club *looking* good too: That's right. It's *clean* sperm! Your sperm is

literally washed clean of all the extraneous fluids and plas-
mas and goop it travels in, so now it's "great sperm, less
semen." This is important because, as we discussed in chapter 2, all that seminal fluid is there to protect the sperm from
the hostile environment in the vagina, and let's face it, if you
know you're not going to be shot at, you leave the body armor
at home. So now the "leaner 'n' meaner" sperm can wiggle
their way to their target unencumbered by anything that can
slow them down or get them stuck.

Now you might ask, "How exactly is my sperm washed?"
Hey, why don't you ask me what's at the end of the universe
while you're at it? Even if I do tell you, it's not like you can
actually do anything with the information. All you need to
know is that you give the lab a fresh sample, and they take
care of the rest. (Fine—it involves spinning it around really
fast. I told you it wasn't important.) As for the actual "hows"
and "heretofores" of giving the sperm, there's a whole chapter later that's all about the proper etiquette of sample collection (Sperm-A-Lot).

Needless to say, this process has to be timed perfectly for
it to achieve maximum effectiveness, and your doctor will
treat it with the precision of a NASA launch. He'll check the
progress of your wife's (now-stimulated) ovulation with a
couple of ultrasound examinations, searching for that perfect launch window. When he determines everything looks
good, he gives the go order, you drop off your payload, the lab
preps it, and boom, up it goes. From that point on it's just a
waiting game to see if your small wiggly astronauts complete
their mission and rendezvous with your wife's waiting egg.

Godspeed, gentlemen!

"OKAY, CHEWIE, WE'RE
JUMPING TO HYPERSTIMULATION!"

Alright, let's be honest; sometimes you need more than just a little help. While Clomid may work for some women, others may need something a little stronger to get the old juices flowing. Actually, something a *lot* stronger. After all, you wouldn't go hunting elephants with just a Daisy air rifle, right? (Not that I'd ever advocate actually hunting elephants— I can't even bring myself to buy Ivory soap, for crying out loud!) It's at this point that a cry goes out: "This is a job for *gonadotropins!*"

Granted, it doesn't exactly trip off the tongue, but gonadotropins are the next rung up on the fertility treatment ladder. These are highly purified versions of LH and FSH, manufactured under many different names, which are injected into your wife in order to stimulate her natural hormone production. Your doctor may prescribe these injections to be given daily for two weeks in a controlled effort to hyperstimulate her ovaries so that they produce more eggs than her natural gonadotropins would normally allow her to make. This technique has therefore been given the incredibly clever name of *controlled ovarian hyperstimulation* (COH). Oh, those wacky scientists!

"Hold on a sec," I hear you ask. "You're saying my wife needs to go to the doctor every day for two weeks just to get an injection?" No, not at all. This is something she gets to do at home—or more precisely, something *you* get to do to her at home. Now before you freak out, read the chapter on giving injections, and you might just change your mind. If you don't, well, I suppose there's the coward's way out: Let her give herself the shots while you put on a dress and weep quietly in the corner. We'll talk about all that stuff later.

But do know that your wife will still have to go to the doctor fairly frequently throughout the two weeks she will be on this medication. The doctor will be taking regular ultrasounds and blood tests in order to make sure she's not *over*stimulating, i.e., growing too many follicles too quickly. That's what folks in the fertility business call a "bad thing."

THIS HORMONE WAS BROUGHT TO YOU BY THE LETTER "PEE"

As we near the end of this section, I'll leave you with this little factoid: Did you know that gonadotropins can be made one of two ways?

1. **Recombinant gonadotropins** (a.k.a. The Cool Scientific Way): The DNA of various gonadotropins are injected into Chinese hamster ovary cells, causing the cells to change and to begin to create various gonadotropins of their own accord.

2. **Urinary gonadotropins:** A lab harvests a raw protein from the urine of menopausal women.

Now I see you making a disgusted face and saying, "Hold up! You mean, I'm either going to be injecting my wife with mutated hamster cells or old lady pee? That's a hell of a choice! Besides, what's the difference?" Answer to question number one is "Yes you are." (Though, with the old lady pee, it's all been highly distilled and purified and all that good drug company stuff, so it's not as if it's coming straight out of Rue McClanahan and into your wife.)

As for the answer to the second question, recombinant gonadotropins have only FSH in them, whereas the urinary gonadotropins contain both FSH and LH, so you obviously get more bang for your buck with the latter.

Studies done by the American Society for Reproductive Medicine have shown that there's almost no difference in the pregnancy rates if you use one versus the other, but a 2005 study at Tel Aviv University did conclude that women who might be susceptible to *ovarian hyperstimulation syndrome* (OHSS—we'll talk about that later) have less of a chance for complications with the urine-based gonadotropins. In any case, your doctor will help you figure out which one is best for you.

C'MON, GIMME JUST ONE MORE SHOT

As the two-week hyperstimulation cycle nears its end and the time for the IUI approaches, there's still *one more* shot that needs to be given—a special gonadotropin called *human chorionic gonadotropin* (hCG), a.k.a. the "trigger shot." It's similar to LH, but this is the shot that matures all the eggs she has now grown as well as signals all of her eggs to release from her ovaries, at which point they start floating down her fallopian tubes to hook up with your nice clean sperm during the IUI.

When you begin this protocol, you need to keep your schedule free and clear for the next two weeks, because it's up to the doctor when this trigger shot is administered, based on what he sees in the ultrasounds. Once again, it's essential for this whole endeavor to be precisely timed—which could be one reason you always see doctors wearing such nice watches. Another reason could be . . . well, you'll probably figure it out when you get your bill.

Once your doctor likes what he sees and says go, your wife will be instructed to take the shot that very night, and thirty-six hours later, the two of you will find yourself at his practice, (hopefully) making babies!

THE GIFT THAT KEEPS ON GIVING

Now, with an IUI, even though things are timed out, there's still the very real chance that the sperm and egg may just miss one another. After all, it is really dark in there. A technique some fertility doctors may opt for is something called GIFT. (Technically it's *gamete intrafallopian transfer*, but I doubt you'd remember that. I didn't.) With GIFT, the egg is removed from the fallopian tube midjourney, mixed with your sperm, and put right back where it was—kind of like setting the two up on a blind date. Is it a guarantee for fertilization? I'll answer that question with another question: How many blind dates did you have that actually worked out?

In all truthfulness, the advancement of reproductive technology in the last few years has relegated this one to the dustbin of ART history, but it can still be used in some cases, such as when the religion of the parents doesn't allow for fertilization outside of the mother's body.

WORKING WITH HORMONES?
WHAT COULD POSSIBLY GO WRONG?

So, you want to hear the downside of this one too, huh? Fine, Negative Ned. Well, probably the biggest one is the risk of overstimulation. This can lead to a very serious condition called ovarian hyperstimulation syndrome (OHSS). I know; it sounds almost the same as controlled ovarian hyperstimulation. But there's a big difference in that one little word: *controlled*.

If too much hormone is released into the body, and too many egg follicles are formed, they could become "leaky," which is exactly what it sounds like. As they leak, the excess fluid builds up in her abdomen—which is, if you haven't guessed, another one of those "bad things." If untreated, this has the very real possibility of leading to some nasty complications, including kidney failure. Before you get all excited, your doctor will be carefully monitoring your wife—specifically watching out for things like this—but if at any point he's not around and your wife starts complaining about feeling *really* bloated, is nauseous, has diarrhea, is unable to urinate, etc., call your doctor. Really. Do *not* start the whole "Me proud man! Can protect wife. Me need no help from puny medical professional!" thing here. Two good rules of thumb when dealing with any potential problems are:

1. *Don't* feel like you need to take care of problems yourself. You most likely have no idea what you're talking about and are probably quoting something you heard on an *ER* rerun two months ago.

2. *Don't* feel like you're disturbing your doctor when you need to have a question answered—ever. It's what he's there for, and, quite frankly, his knowledge is the reason you're paying him the equivalent of a luxury vacation for two—including room service and a couple of those ridiculously overpriced pay-per-view movies. (Twelve dollars to watch *Confessions of a Shopaholic*? Come on!)

Besides, if there *does* turn out to be anything wrong, calling your doctor's attention to the problem means he might be able to catch it and do something about it that much sooner.

The other caveat when playing around with gonadotropins is pretty much the same as the one regarding Clomid: Beware the possibility of multiple births. Only difference is that unlike Clomid, which is designed to produce only one or two eggs, gonadotropins could lead to your wife popping out a lot more—like a whole litter. Oh, yeah, we're talking the whole enchilada: quads or quints or even—hey, what *is* the shorthand for six kids? "Sexes"? Wait, that doesn't sound right at all . . .

Remember, when you're doing an IUI, you're basically throwing sperm all up in there and however many eggs they find floating around could also be the same number of kids you eventually end up with. Gonadotropins give you a *lot* of eggs, so . . .

JUST DO IT—*AGAIN*?

So the two of you tried the Clomid. Nothing happened. Then you moved up to the IUIs. Nope. IUIs plus gonadotropins? Nada. But, being the doer that you are, you try again. And again. And again.

I don't know what your time frame is for having children, or what your finances look like, but the one thing all of these procedures have in common is that they take time and money. And lots of each.

If you think about it time-wise, you can only do one fertility treatment a month—duh—and usually it's recommended you take at least a month or two off in between, just to give her body a rest from the medication. (Plus—and this is never mentioned by the doctor—it's good for your own sanity to take some time off too. Believe me. She ain't gonna be a pussycat when she's on that hormone cocktail.)

Anyway, I'm truly, sincerely hoping one of the above protocols works for you, but in the unhappy event that it doesn't, even after repeated tries, the two of you may eventually find yourselves running out of time, money, or patience. It's at this point you might want to consider moving on to what I like to think of as the Big Daddy of all fertility treatments: IVF.

SIX

IVF: It's Very Frustrating!

*C*ongratulations! Nothing's worked!

If you're even bothering to read this chapter, I'll wager that the two of you are at the end of your rope, what with all the pills and shots and IUIs and maybe even a Santeria priest or two, but even with all that—wow, how can I put this delicately?—you've crapped out.

You know what? I realize this may ring hollow, but you really shouldn't feel that bad. If you learn one thing from this book, let it be that fertility treatments are not a one-size-fits-all kind of thing. Everyone's got their own issues, and what works for some couples doesn't work for others. There are always going to be some problems that take a little more work to overcome. You want some modern Zen? Then meditate on this: There's a reason they make extrastrength stain remover.

Pretty deep, huh? Believe it or not I came up with that little gem while I was doing the laundry.

If every couple were able to get pregnant easily, even with Clomid and IUIs, they would never have had to come up with IVF, which might very well turn out to be your golden ticket. And more importantly, I'd be a whole chapter short in this book and I'd have to fill in this space with old stories of when

I was in Indian Guides or something. And trust me, *nobody* wants to hear those.

So now you're here, gingerly dipping your toes into the highest of high-tech fertility treatments: IVF. In vitro fertilization, a.k.a. the test-tube baby. (Although actually that's a misnomer, seeing as everything happens in a petri dish—but I guess not enough people know what a petri dish is, and nothing screams "Science!" like a test tube. See, in the end it's all about the marketing.)

As the old saying goes, "Forewarned is forearmed," so it's my job to make sure you know as much as you can about this kind of treatment. It's definitely not for everyone, and if you do end up going down this road, you're in for one hell of a ride.

JOIN THE CLUB!

Couples who go through IVF are part of a very exclusive club—granted, not exactly the kind of club people are beating down the gates to join, but exclusive nonetheless. Only about 2 percent of couples dealing with infertility actually do IVF, so it really is, under normal circumstances, the technique of last resort.

There are usually only a few reasons you might be in the IVF boat:

1. If your wife's reproductive system is compromised (e.g., if there is a blockage in the fallopian tubes or endometriosis occurring).

2. If your wife has reached an age where the quality of her eggs has deteriorated to the point where a normal conception is impossible.

3. If you've got some really poor-quality sperm or a low sperm count.

But if IVF is thought of as the fertility treatment method of last resort, it can also be said that it's the method with the greatest amount of control, as every last detail—from the timing of the egg growth to which individual sperm penetrates the egg—can be manipulated for the greatest effect. Ain't science cool?

YOU HAVE NO IDEA ABOUT
WHAT YOU HAVE NO IDEA ABOUT

As you start reading through this chapter, there will come a point, probably in the next couple of pages, where you'll say to yourself, "Wow, there sure are a lot of similarities between IVF and IUI." You'd be right. After which there's a good chance you'll start believing that since you were smart enough to figure that one out, you really don't need to read through to the end of the chapter. After all, it's pretty much the same thing with different initials, right?

Do not, I repeat do not not read this chapter all the way through—which is the double-negative way of saying *read it*. I'm telling you right now that you haven't the slightest clue as to what IVF is about. If you did, you wouldn't be reading this book—and more importantly, your wife wouldn't have bought it for you. That's always a nice big hint that she wants you to know something she's sure you don't—like when she tucks that issue of *Consumer Reports* comparing new washer/dryers into your briefcase.

Now, the good news is that the whole IVF process *makes sense*, at least in a logical, progressive kind of way. This is really, really important, because all in all, this is how we men think. When we find ourselves faced with a problem, we step back, take a look at what the job will entail, and then find a logical way to solve it. IVF is a very straightforward idea that progresses in a very easy-to-understand pattern. As I said, that's the good news.

The bad news is that logic has almost nothing to do with *going through* IVF. You've no doubt heard of the proverbial "emotional roller coaster"? Well, Six Flags ain't got nothing on the ride you're gonna get out of this thing. You're going to be white-knuckling the safety bar and throwing up on every single drop and S-turn, and before it's over you'll swear the track you're riding on was designed by the sickest, most sadistic son of a bitch on two legs.

But before I go and scare you too much with all this "emotions" crap, let's look at what the whole process of IVF entails. Then you can be scared.

HOLD THAT ORDER OF EGGS, WILL YA?

Okay, you like riddles? Try this one on: In order to grow her eggs, you must first stop her eggs from growing.

Mind scrambler, right? I hear you saying, "But how can you have eggs if you have no eggs, but if you need eggs you don't have but..." And then smoke starts pouring out of your ears and you shut off. Or maybe you're just confused. Either way, I'm here to help.

Believe it or not, that's actually the logic behind the first step of IVF. Your wife needs to stop producing eggs, and guess what? You're going to help her do it.

See, with IVF, as with most of these fertility treatments, timing is *everything*. So much so that the doctor doesn't want to leave the slightest bit of biological mischief to chance. So the first thing he does is begin a series of injections of a drug most commonly called Lupron, which is technically referred to as a *gonadotropin-releasing hormone agonist*. Now, if you're like me, I'm fairly certain the first word you zeroed in on was "agonist." Don't worry—it has nothing to do with pain. At least not yet.

An agonist is a drug designed to elicit a specific reaction in a specific cell. In this case, the specific activity is to shut off your wife's ovulation cycle. Poof. Puts it right to sleep. This way, she won't be making eggs until the doctor is ready for her to begin making eggs. Neat, huh? Otherwise, your doctor would be running around like a maniac, trying to find every egg she creates, and then trying to catch them before they release, effectively turning a highly precise, delicate medical procedure into an episode of *I Love Lucy*.

You might have noticed that your wife will have been taking the birth control pill for about a month before starting the Lupron. Why? Because it helps regulate her period, which in turn helps her and her doctor know when to start the medication.

About one week before she's scheduled to get her period, you'll start injecting your wife with the Lupron, which will stop her from any early ovulation, as well as help the doctor set up a controlled IVF schedule for her.

And yes, just in case you didn't read that last sentence (or even if you did read the last sentence but pretended to "accidentally" skip over it), I'll repeat: *You* will be the one to give your wife the shots. Trust me, you'll get over the "Dude! Gross!" factor pretty quickly, it's not particularly difficult, and more to the point, what kind of man would have his own wife give herself injections?

I'll tell you what kind of a man—a total and complete bastard kind of a man, that's who! And what the hell kid wants to say he has a total and complete *bastard* for a father? So yeah, you'll give her those shots, and you'll smile while you're doing it.

Besides, you being the one doing it means you can honestly say you pushed at least *something* inside of your wife to help conceive the baby!

MORE ON THIS SITUATION
AS IT DEVELOPS

So it goes on like this for about a week: You give her the Lupron shots, she complains about the Lupron shots, says you're not doing it right (even if you are), and so on. At the end of the week, she gets her period . . . well, sort of. Technically, because of the Lupron, nothing much comes out, but *she* knows it's happening, and it's the trigger for the next stage.

The next morning, your wife will go back into your fertility doctor's office for more blood tests and ultrasounds. They'll check her hormone levels to make sure they are where they should be, and the ultrasound checks her ovaries to be sure the Lupron put everything to sleep and that the follicles are ready to go for round two.

So later that afternoon, she'll get a call from the office that tells her it's time to make the donuts, which, for those of you who don't know classic TV commercials, is really obscure code for "Time to wake up the eggs and get this baby-making show on the road!"

(Oh, yeah, and you have to give her a lot more shots now, too. Man, is she gonna hate you.)

WAKEY WAKEY, EGGS AND . . .
YEAH, PRETTY MUCH JUST THE EGGS

As with almost everything fertility related, at this point there's good news and bad news. The good news: You get to give your wife a lot less Lupron, about half of what you were giving her for the last week. The bad news? You're going to be making up the difference with two new drugs, one of which is going to sting like a sum'bitch. (IMPORTANT NOTE: If you know what's good for you, you will *not* tell her that last part. I'm just giving you a heads-up so you can brace yourself for the inevitable rage that'll no doubt come your way. More on that later in the chapter on giving shots.)

This is how it will go down: After your wife gets her tests back, the doctor will decide what it's going to take in order to get her eggs up and at 'em, and then prescribe the right combination of gonadotropins, (a.k.a. *follicle stimulating medications*). This is harder than it sounds: Too much medication might result in a big batch of low-quality eggs, as well as the possibility of ovarian hyperstimulation syndrome.

There's an underlying irony to the fact that all of these methods fall under the term "ART." A critical concept you really need to understand—and something you will find repeated throughout this book—is that while IVF is most definitely a science, it's also an *art*, as in the creative kind of art. This is the point where you truly learn if your doctor is a Picasso or just that guy at the swap meet who paints Led Zeppelin album art on black velvet. (I'm not ragging on either Zeppelin or black velvet, mind you, but there's a time and a place ...)

So now it's up to your doctor to come up with a cocktail of drugs to stimulate your wife's ovaries into producing eggs—and not just any eggs, but good eggs. After all, you wouldn't want your breakfast omelet to come from a bunch of cracked, drippy eggs, would you? Okay, maybe that wasn't the greatest example, but the point is still valid, and there really aren't a lot of analogies to draw on when it comes to eggs, you know?

There are a few different types of drugs your doctor may prescribe, either alone or in combination. These can go under the names Menopur, Follistim, Luveris, Gonal-F, Bravelle, and Repronex. Some are the urinary-based gonadotropins (Menopur, Repronex) and some (Follistim, Luveris) are the recombinant kind (both of these gonadotropin types are covered in more detail in chapter 5). Since each fertility patient is different, your doctor will be helping you determine which are the right drugs for you.

On a side note, I love the names of these drugs. It's like they were all thought up by the same guys who decide what to name new car models: "How about 'Maxima'? It's not a real word, but sounds like it could be!" I picture the scientists at the lab having spent all their energy actually inventing the drug, and then when it was all over and it came time to name it, they just said, "Oh, screw that—we're exhausted! Fine, you want a name? It stimulates the follicles—call it 'Follistim.' Yeah, sounds nice and science-y!"

This is also the DIY portion of the process, where you get to play mad scientist mixing it up in the lab. See, giving Lupron is relatively easy (for you, anyway): You pull it out of the vial with the syringe and then put it into your wife. What did I say? Easy. But these new medications—these gonadotropins—well, they're another matter entirely, mostly because of the way they're made.

Each "serving" of these drugs comes in two vials: one saline solution, one drug powder. Your job is to mix them together, and then give her the shot. Again, do not panic. It's not really that difficult. I mean sure, at first it can be a little intimidating; after all, unless you have experience running a meth lab, mixing drugs can be a little tricky. I promise you'll get the hang of it. But one caveat: No matter how well you do it, as far as your wife is concerned, you won't do it right. Ever. It's not an insult, but more of a "giving up control" thing she's trying to deal with. It's okay. It happened to all of us. It'll happen to you. Roll with it.

THE RAGE AND PAIN
WILL MAKE YOUR WIFE INSANE

So you inject her with this drug cocktail for the next week, give or take a few days. During this time, she'll be going in to see the doctor every other day, all the while getting poked and prodded, bled and ultrasounded in order to make sure her eggs are developing on schedule, but not too fast. Along the way, your doctor may adjust the medication amounts up or down, based on what he thinks is necessary. (NOTE: That fact doesn't really matter to you, except that the more medication your wife is given, the more she thinks you're messing it up.)

As the week wears on, and the protocol draws to a close, pretty soon you'll notice that your wife is going to the fertility clinic for tests every day. Even if you don't notice, you'll know it's happening because she'll be mentioning it a lot, as in: "Oh, so you want to know why there's no dinner? How about because I've been too busy getting stuck with needles and having cold electronic things shoved up inside of my hoo-ha every damn morning!"

At this point she may or may not go on and refer to you as "an insensitive prick who has absolutely no idea what I'm going through." To which you'll be tempted to say, "Yeah I do, because you won't stop complaining about it for one second!" My best advice? Resist that temptation. Resist it like a triathlete resists pie.

You *won't* say that kind of stuff out loud, *ever*, and I'll give you two good reasons why: 1) quite frankly, we guys really don't have any idea what she's going through, and 2) with all of those megahormones raging through her system, she could pick you up and tear you in half lengthwise before you could even open your stupid yap to apologize.

Word is truth.

Yeah, it's at this point in the protocol that these last few weeks of hormone treatments really start catching up with her. Under normal circumstances, she may be the sweetest thing on two feet, just skipping along picking flowers and petting puppies, but that all's going to come to a screeching halt, my friend.

In our case, my normally mellow wife, Julie, suddenly found herself in a cascade of emotions, alternately feeling angry, hungry, weepy—and all the rest of Snow White's dwarves' evil twins—and generally out of control, and guess who got a front-row seat! It's like a big fun preview of a pregnancy all squeezed into three weeks. Yay for me. There are, of course, many ways of trying to deal with all of these hormonal swings—some of which might even work. I'll cover these in the upcoming chapter. Trust me, I'm here to help.

PULL 'EM OUT! PULL 'EM OUT! WAAAY OUT!

So by this time, if all goes right, her eggs should be nice and, well, woken. When the doctor has determined that a suitable number of eggs have reached a mature state and size, he'll make the call, both figuratively and literally, and give you the good news: It's time to retrieve those eggs and start putting the F into IVF.

Okay, the doctor likes what he sees. Good for you! Now we have to get those bad boys out of your wife and stick them into a petri dish in the lab. To do that, we need to pull the fire alarm and evacuate the building. And how is that done? Why, by giving her another shot, of course. Oh, yeah, your wife is gonna *love* you when you're done with all of this!

This time the drug of choice is a little mixture called hCG (human chorionic gonadotropin), which you may remember is also used in IUI. It's a synthetic hormone that acts as a trigger, basically telling your wife to ovulate on demand. And since it's such a momentous shot, you get to give it in a momentous way: Unlike the subcutaneous shots you've been giving your wife in the skin above her stomach, this bad boy needs to be given *intramuscularly*—and if you don't know what that means ... well, in the immortal words of the *Newlywed Game* urban legend, "That'd be in the butt, Bob."

You'll get the call from the fertility clinic about thirty-two to thirty-six hours before harvesting time, and yet again timing is everything. They literally count backward from your appointment thirty-two to thirty-six hours, and that's pretty much exactly when you *must* give her the shot.

Consider this fair warning: If you both get too engrossed in *Law and Order*, and just at the moment the DA is about to spring that one piece of damning evidence that will reduce the cocky defendant into a quivering pile of goo, you turn to each other and realize, "Aw, crap! Weren't we supposed to do the shot a half hour ago?" Hey, guess what? You're screwed. Like I said before, this is precision stuff. My best advice? Set alarms around the house. A lot of them. Get creative; your microwave and cell phones have alarms too. I don't give a crap if they beep, ring, honk, or play *Clair de Lune* in B-flat minor; it's your job to set them to go off at the right time. Do that, and you'll go a long way toward avoiding any potential problems.

When the time comes, give her the shot, listen to her complain about it for a while (with a smile on your face, of course), and then . . . well, you wait.

FERTILIZE 'ER

Two days later, you've taken the morning off of work and you and your wife are sitting in the waiting room at your fertility clinic. She's going to be nervous, with good reason: She's about to go through something your doctor calls an *aspiration cycle*, or just "aspiration." It's a pretty word; it sounds nice and light and airy. What does it mean? Well, it means that under light (but still general) anesthetic, your wife will have a long, thin needle inserted into her vagina, up to her ovaries, and each mature egg will be carefully plucked from its individual follicle (i.e., aspirated), sucked up into the syringe, and gently placed into a petri dish, awaiting eventual fertilization. She'll have to spend about an hour in recovery, just to make sure there aren't any postoperative complications or bleeding.

You, on the other hand, will go off into the next room to masturbate.

Okay, there's a little more to it than that, seeing as this isn't your average "get up in the morning and rub one out" session, but all of the details of your chore will be covered in chapter 7.

So there we have it: her egg, your sperm. Let's make us a baby!

EMBRYOS CHECK IN, AND, HOPEFULLY, THEY'LL CHECK OUT

When a movie is made, sure, all the actors and directors and well, sometimes writers, get all the attention and accolades, but really, without the people behind the scenes doing important work, like lighting the scenes, getting the film to and from the set, editing the shots, and creating special effects, nothing would get done. Without these people, *Lord of the Rings* would just be a bunch of people running around New Zealand playing a big game of Dungeons and Dragons.

Similarly, while the doctors and the nurses get all of the face time with you and your wife, and thus get the credit for the fertility process (and rightly so), we can't forget the boys and girls in the lab, whose names you probably don't know and who also deserve a huge part of the credit, since if it wasn't for them, your genetic material would just be sitting idly in test tubes, looking around forlorn, wondering what to do next.

But what happens in the lab? How do they mix the sperm and egg together? Do they get grossed out handling all those fluids? I can't answer that last one, but as for the first two:

The first thing you need to know is that within minutes of collecting your wife's egg and your sperm, both are quickly whisked off to the lab. (NOTE: This is one of the maybe two instances in your life when you can actually use the term "whisked off" and not be beaten up.) Her eggs are observed and graded according to size and maturity, and your sperm is washed and stress tested like little fighter pilot trainees until only the hardiest, best-looking sperm are left. Hey, you're spending a lot of money to have this kid, so might as well make him or her the best you can, right?

So, on average, out of the millions (well, give or take, depending on your particular situation) of sperm you give to the lab, only about a hundred thousand will make it past the velvet rope to swim around in the petri dish with her egg. Now while in the real world this is what we'd consider a serious "sausage party," it's an ideal situation in the fertility world, as it allows the sperm easier access to the egg. And remember, one industrious sperm is all we're looking for here.

Once the egg has been fertilized, it is placed into an incubator and allowed to, well, incubate. After a couple of days, the lab techs open it up again in order to see if any of the eggs have actually been fertilized. If so, mazel tov! You've got yourself an embryo! Actually, you can have yourself a whole bunch of embryos, but that doesn't necessarily mean it's great news. What you need to realize is that just because an egg has been fertilized, and you have an embryo, that doesn't guarantee it's automatically going to develop into a fine strapping young man who goes All State in three sports yet still has time to clean out the garage on Saturdays. (I say if you're gonna dream, dream big.)

Consider this example: Back in college, we all knew that one guy who one day decided to use all of his God-given intelligence and industriousness to try to grow pot. Adopting the mantra of "if you grow it, they will come," he went ahead and spent tons of money, set up a state-of-the-art hydroponics nursery in his dorm room with equipment he swiped from the chem labs, and planted a whole lotta seeds. What happened? Did that guy end up becoming the all-powerful weed mogul for the entire dorm he dreamed of being? Unless you happened to go to school with Tony Montana, I'm going to assume the answer would be a big fat no.

See, even though conditions may have been perfect theoretically, and his seeds may have even fertilized, in the end, some chance error—maybe a variation of temperature, too much or too little light, whatever—stopped his herbal garden from taking root and growing. (Oh, and on top of that he probably got his dumb stoner ass thrown out of school too.)

Strangely tangential allegories about collegiate weed farming aside, when it comes right down to making embryos, sometimes a lack of viability can be explained by something as simple as an immature egg, or as complex and statistically freaky weird as two sperm entering the egg at the exact same time. The embryologists are looking for embryos that fertilize and seem like they have the ability to "go the distance." Then they grade them, pretty much the same way the USDA grades a piece of steak.

Needless to say, what you're looking for is the prime-cut, A-grade New York sirloin, versus that D-minus-grade, "Eh, sell it to the school cafeteria; those dopey kids won't know the difference" mystery meat.

Unlike that delicious cut of meat, however, grading embryos has less to do with lean marbling and more to do with the way the cells divide. What embryologists are looking for is the smooth, even division of cells, with very little *fragmentation* (uneven, ugly, broken-off little bits and pieces that can hang around the edges of divided cells). This is the one time that a basic, fundamental tenet of the male brain applies in fertility: If it doesn't look good, we don't want it.

After the embryos have spent three days in the incubators, the embryologists want to see ones that have already divided into at least six to eight cells, all of which look nice and symmetrical to one another. By day five, these cells have (hopefully) divided and divided again and again, until we're looking at a mass made up of around sixty-four to one hundred cells. When you have one of these, you are officially in possession of what's called a *blastocyst*.

Yes, I know; it has the words "blast" and "cyst" in it, so to our untrained man-ears it sounds like it'd be bad. And explosive. In actuality, having a blastocyst is the exact *opposite* of bad (which, according to my edition of *Roget's Thesaurus*, happens to be "good"). In IVF, you're constantly looking for the "good"; therefore, you want those blastocysts. You want a whole lot of 'em.

Why? Because by the time an embryo can be called a blastocyst, it is considered mature enough to actually implant itself into the uterus. In fact, half of its cells are what will eventually become a baby, and half are what will become the placenta.

What do you do if you have lots and lots of good embryos? One popular option is something called *cryopreservation*, where the embryos are frozen a la Buck Rodgers and then kept in cold storage at the clinic. These embryos can then be thawed out again at a later date if you want to go for another

IVF implantation treatment, or they can be given to another couple if you wish (through a process called embryo donation, which I'll discuss in more detail in chapter 10).

Now it's time for another edition of Good News/Bad News. The good news: For fertility doctors, this is the stage at which the embryo stands the best chance of successfully implanting. The bad news: It may very well turn out that you won't get to the point where you have blastocysts to implant. It all depends on how many embryos you actually have.

Now if it happens that you hit the IVF jackpot and you have something like ten embryos fertilize in the lab within the first three days, then what the hell, go ahead and wait a couple of extra days to see which ones turn out to develop into your best blastocysts, and then pop those suckers inside and watch 'em take root.

If, however, the first seventy-two hours roll by and you only have two, three, or four embryos that successfully fertilize, then that annoying old idiom "beggars can't be choosers" suddenly starts making a whole lot of sense to you. With so few options, your doctor will most likely do the fertility version of what is known in poker as "going all in," and put *every embryo* back inside her, in the hopes that at least one will make it to the blastocyst stage in her uterus and implant. This technique has been given the very complex name of the *three-day implantation cycle*, as opposed to the *five-day implantation cycle*. Damned complicated medical jargon!

Now, for some couples, the idea of having their children mixed up in a lab, or sitting in a petri dish for too long, just doesn't sound appealing, or they may have some religious or cultural objections to the idea. For those people, there is a slightly different technique, considered the older cousin to GIFT (see chapter 5), which is known as ZIFT or *zygote intrafallopian transfer.*

In this procedure, the lab makes sure the sperm fertilizes the egg, creating what's called a zygote (which is really just a fancy-schmancy name for a fertilized egg). This zygote is then placed directly back into the fallopian tube as soon as possible in the hopes it will travel down and implant in the uterus as nature intended. Note that this is different from a three-day transfer, in which the zygotes are allowed to develop into embryos first, and then transferred directly into the uterus to implant.

Now, for obvious reasons, five-day transfers are better (you get the better-developed and higher-quality embryos, and thus a better chance of implantation in the uterus), but don't go and freak out if you don't have one. If and when they implant, embryos transferred after three days have a nearly identical chance of resulting in pregnancy as the five-day ones.

That's not to say there aren't other issues you may have to deal with if you go the three-day route. As is the case with the use of Clomid or gonadotropins, one possible result from the "throw it against the uterus and see what sticks" method is an increased chance of "multiple births." It makes sense, right? After all, since the doctors can't be that selective about which fertilized eggs are used, the more they do put in, the more there are that have a chance to take root and grow.

To illustrate, I'll put it in financial terms, since all of us have money—well, at least we all *did* before we started fertility treatments.

Anyway, common wisdom has it that the more diversified your investment portfolio is, the less chance you have of taking a full-on hit in the shorts when something goes wrong. Conversely, it also means the better chance you have of at least one of your stocks doing well. When doctors throw everything into your wife's uterus (in all fairness, they're a *bit* more delicate than that when they perform the transfer procedure—see below), they're thinking, "Well, we can hope that at least one of these embryos will take hold and start developing." You've gotta love that kind of positive thinking!

PGD IN THE USA!

It's at this point in the protocol that you have the option for a fancy little something that we in the know call PGD or *preimplantation genetic diagnosis*. Simply put, they take one cell from the eight or so your embryo has by day three, send it off to a lab, and check for any specific genetic damage. Pretty amazing stuff. This is useful if you have a history of a specific genetic defect running through your family and you want to find out ahead of time if the little nipper will have it or not. Or it's also recommended if your wife is over forty; women of that age tend to have some severe genetic degradation in their ova.

Two things about PGD, though: First of all, it's expensive. When you think about it, it kind of has to be. Do you have any idea how hard it is to pull one cell from an embryo without damaging it, and then decode the DNA in the cell to look for specific indicators of damage or disorders? Well, neither do

I ... but I assume it's really hard. Think about how much you shell out for a mechanic to put a new fuel pump in your car. Now multiply that difficulty level by, oh, say *a billion* (that's a raw guess about the statistics of the thing, but I'm not a math teacher, so you'll have to go with me on this).

The other problem is that you'll need to put together an extensive genetic history of any bad fruit that might be hanging off your family tree for the geneticists to attempt to identify and decode. Depending on your family, this will either be easy or impossible. If you happen to have a mother like mine, who takes great joy in having recorded every detail of the Wolfe family saga—from the shtetls of eastern Europe to the suburbs of Southern California—like some sort of Jewish Alex Haley, well, then you're golden. If not, it is obviously going to be quite a bit harder for you.

Your doctor and wife have much more information about PGD, and while it's obviously not something you necessarily *have* to do, it's always nice to know you have the option.

Okay, so we're assuming you now have your eight to one hundred cell embryos doing laps in a lab dish. Great! Now all we need to do is get them into your wife ...

TAKE THE LOCAL TO THE VAGINA, THEN TRANSFER AT THE UTERUS ...

It doesn't matter whether it's the third or fifth day after retrieval, the day you go back to your fertility doctor for the embryo transfer is one pretty intense day. Oh, sure, you'll be all macho and offer up a strong shoulder for your wife to lean on, but deep down, you're just as nervous as she is. After all, you've been a part of this process from the beginning, and this is the moment of truth—or at least the moment before the moment of truth, and for the most part, well, it's out of your hands now.

Think about when you were in school and you were assigned a research paper. It took weeks and weeks to do all of the painstaking research, write your drafts, type it up, and then finally turn it in to the teacher. Then it hits you: Once that research paper leaves your hands, from that point on it's all up to the good graces of your teacher—which, soon after becoming a high school teacher myself, I quickly realized depends entirely on whether or not I've had strong enough coffee that particular morning.

When you and your wife go through fertility treatments, especially one as drawn out and complex as IVF, it can be very difficult to give up control. You spend your adult life making decisions about what you're going to do: You decide where you're going to eat, which crappy movie you're going to spend twelve bucks on even though you never wanted to see it in the first place, and then you decide whom to complain about it to afterward. But now, here's this thing where, after you make the decision to do it, it's out of your hands pretty much as soon as your penis is in your hands in the specimen room.

When Julie and I went through our first embryo transfer (all told we went through three, never even having gotten to the point of transfer during our first IVF cycle), of course we were nervous. Our situation was that we were on a three-day protocol, we had three embryos to put in, and from what our doctor was telling us, they looked just "fine." You don't want "fine." You want "good" or "great" or "quick, get the *New England Journal of Medicine* on the phone for this one!" Basically, we were going into the Super Bowl with our second string.

Being a man, I had on my game face the entire drive over to the clinic, reassuring Julie that everything would be okay. "Pshht! No problem! People do this all the time!" Since she was all read up on the subject, and had way more factual information at her disposal than I did, she was nervously quoting me success statistics about how low the chances are that this would work with our particular circumstances, our ages, our previous lack of success, our zodiac signs, and any other demographic we could possibly be broken down into.

Showing the exact same ill-conceived bravado I use when I challenge my eighteen-year-old students to pick-up basketball games, I continued to assure her that there was nothing to worry about. Needless to say, I had no idea what I was talking about, and more to the point I had no idea what they were going to do to (and with) her. All I knew was that in this situation I wasn't going to be dunked on in front of everyone. Man, that hurts.

Now, it turns out that the actual procedure begins earlier that day, before you even get there. Over in the lab, those highly skilled technicians take the embryos that are about to be transferred and do a procedure called *assisted hatching* (AH). What happens here is the tech makes a tiny hole in the outer shell, or *zona*, of the embryo with a drop of acid. The idea behind this is that if there's already a clearly marked EXIT sign there in the egg, the embryo inside will push on out a lot more easily, and then separate from the egg and implant itself in the uterus. Makes perfect sense, right?

The transfer process itself is a lot less complicated than the retrieval. In fact, it only takes fifteen minutes, and this time you don't get to go off and masturbate while it's being done (which can be a good or bad thing, depending on your particular proclivities).

The only obvious downside is that until it's over, your wife is going to be sitting there with a full bladder, and thus not in the best of moods. Why? Long story short, a full bladder presses up on the uterus, which makes it easier for the doctor to do his business. Good for the doctor, bad for your wife, who's going to be feeling every single pothole and speed bump on the drive down to the doctor's office. And you could be a real dick about it like I was and constantly make jokes about rainstorms, warm hot tubs, and waterfalls, but I wouldn't recommend it.

So, once you get to your doctor's office, you and your wife are led into a sterile room where your doctor, an embryologist, and a nurse or two are waiting for you. Your wife then jumps up onto the exam table and puts her legs up in those metal stirrups you always play with when you're all alone in the exam rooms. Admit it.

Next, the doctor turns on the overhead klieg light, takes a catheter loaded with your embryos, then, using an ultrasound machine, slides it into her vagina all the way up to her uterus, and bam—the embryos are deposited. Okay, less of a bam and more like a soft squish. And then . . . well, nothing. That's it. They check to make sure the catheter is empty, have your wife lie there for another twenty minutes or so, and then you go home and start praying.

So this prompts the question, "Hey, I didn't see anything about the husband in that description. Why do I have to be there?" Well, if I really have to spell it out for you, you're supposed to be there for encouragement, to hold your wife's hand, stroke her forehead, and tell her everything is going great and that she's amazing. At least that's the idealized version. The truth? It's kind of hard to play cheerleader when all you can see is your doctor's head underneath the sheet between your wife's legs (although then again, depending on what you're into . . .).

So what happens when you get back home? Your doctor will probably recommend that your wife stay off her feet for one to three days. There's no scientific evidence that it helps implantation one way or another; it's more just a grace period for having had a big needle stuck up her hoo-ha. It would be a nice thing for you to be extra attentive and loving during this time. Oh, and you should know about the two big no-nos during the next couple of days: no strenuous exercise, and no sex.

I'm assuming you see that the exercise one is pretty self-evident. You don't want her kickboxing while you're trying to get your little guy (or girl) to implant inside her. Yes, I know she still looks bloated from all of the fertility drugs, and yes I know you'd like her to be the svelte goddess you went to Cancun with that one time, and you'd love to see her come to bed in something other than that oversize Cowboys T-shirt and boxers, but think of it this way: At least you won't be as surprised if and when she gets pregnant and puts on the baby weight.

The other thing we need to talk about is sex. As in, no sex. As in, "Oh, crap! Still no sex?" Hey, cut her some slack; it's not just to mess with your head. There's a damn good reason for it. See, when a woman orgasms, her uterus contracts. Now normally, this is a good thing, as it helps move sperm up inside of her and that much closer to her eggs. But remember, you've already done that part—or at least your doctor has. If her uterus goes through contractions at this point, you run the risk of having it tighten up when it needs to be nice and relaxed for the embryo to implant, and that's not what we want. No one wants to move into his California dream house during an earthquake, you know?

Listen, if it makes you feel better, just tell yourself that since you always deliver so much pleasure to your wife during lovemaking, giving her so much ecstasy at this crucial point would be detrimental to the whole fertility process; so out of kindness you'll hold off using your supreme erotic powers for the time being, and deny her that earth-shaking orgasm. (Wives, if you're reading this part of the book, I'm asking you nicely to stop snickering before he asks you what's so funny. It'll save you a lot of ego stroking later.)

Some of the things she can do when she's home: walk around and pee. If your wife is anything like mine, she'll have a big problem with this second one. For some reason, even having a pretty good grasp of her own anatomy, Julie was convinced beyond a shadow of a doubt that as soon as she sat down on that toilet, the embryos would just fall right out of her and we'd literally be flushing our dreams of parenthood away.

So what should you do if you find this happening? I'll tell you: If the time comes when she becomes irrational and actually starts crying about this, you'll want to sit her down, gently take her hands in yours, look deeply into her eyes, and, in a steady voice, say to her in no uncertain terms these calming words: "ARE YOU CRAZY? YOU CAN'T PEE OUT IMPLANTED EMBRYOS! THE DOCTOR PUT THEM IN YOUR *UTERUS*, NOT YOUR BLADDER! DAMMIT, WOMAN! HAVE YOU *NO* IDEA HOW HUMAN ANATOMY WORKS?" Let me stress, this is what you'll *want* say. You'll want it with every fiber of your being. *Don't*. Don't. Don't. Don't. Just . . . just don't, okay?

Instead, what you should do is gently remind her that the doctor put the embryos deep into her uterus. The "uterus" has nothing to do with "urine," other than that they both start with the letter U. Your wife is going to be afraid. Maybe you'll be afraid too. For better or for worse, and at the risk of being called sexist, a lot of the time it's going to fall upon you, the man, to try to keep both of your moods nice and even, and the two of you hanging onto the good side of sane.

YOU'RE LAYING IT ON PRETTY THICK THERE

Okay, you have the embryos in her uterus, floating around. The goal now is to get them to find a nice place to settle down, make a home, implant, and start growing. Remember that the uterine lining is called the endometrium? If you don't, you should learn that right now, because for the next couple of weeks that word's going to dominate your wife's vocabulary, whether she's talking to her doctor, her friends, or the other

IVF-ers on the online boards (oh, yeah, we'll get to *them* later).

Yep, for the next couple of weeks after the transfer, you and your wife will be on a mission to thicken up that endometrium to the point where no embryo can resist plopping down on there, snuggling in, and growing into a cute little baby. And how does one thicken up an endometrium? Easy: by increasing the amount of progesterone in your wife's system.

As you'll remember, progesterone is a naturally occurring hormone that's meant to thicken up the lining of the uterus and make it sticky enough. And we get the progesterone into her the same we do *everything* in IVF—with more shots, of course!

See, the same drugs your wife takes to increase her egg supply oftentimes deplete her body's store of progesterone. And just in case you weren't sure, yes, this situation is a perfect illustration of irony—or at least a better one than all those lame examples in that Alanis Morissette song. (Sorry, but getting a spoon when you want a knife falls under "bad service," not irony.)

So every night for the next, oh, let's say two weeks or so, you'll be jabbing a big ol' needle into your wife's ass. Now I hear you smiling smugly and saying, "No problem, because I've already been giving her shots throughout this whole thing just like you said to, so there!" That's great, and I applaud your male sensitivity. Unfortunately, I have some bad news: You know those other shots? Mosquitoes. Pin pricks. For this bad boy, you're going to have to mount up on your steed and hold the thing like a lance at a medieval jousting tournament. And just like at one of those tournaments, if you miss or do it wrong, "off with your head." (Not really, but your wife will get super pissed off at you if you screw it up.)

There's also the option of *pessaries,* which are progesterone suppositories your wife could put up inside of her vagina every night. But even if she thinks that's what she wants, she won't use it. By this time in the protocol, Julie was screaming, "No more needles, no more needles!" But after trying to work with this messy, slippery, gooey alternative, she basically walked up to me, dropped her pants, bent over, and said, "Fire away."

Basically for the next couple of weeks, your wife is going to be on a constant mini-PMS: i.e., constipated, nauseous, tired, feeling bloated and irritable—and that's on top of the excruciating anxiety about the upcoming pregnancy test. She's going to be a mess. You're probably not going to be much better, but at least she has the hormones to blame for what she says and does, so it's really, really important that during this final lap you're Johnny-on-the-spot. Try not to take anything she says personally, because believe me, she'll say things. Bad things. Really, really bad things. Things involving your mother and hard drugs and various species of livestock.

Look, it'd be easy to get frustrated and fire back at her, but that's not going to help anyone. What you have to do is focus your energy on making her feel as safe and secure as you can. Your primary job during these crucial two weeks is to be her anchor—even if you're feeling just as adrift as she is.

After all, as long as *you* know the truth about your mother and that goat, that's all that really matters.

I'M ABSOLUTELY, POSITIVELY SORT OF SURE THAT I MAY DEFINITELY BE PREGNANT—OR NOT

By this time, after weeks and weeks of hormone treatments, your wife is really, really in tune with her body; as in she can feel every twinge, twitch, rumble, and cramp—or at least she *thinks* she can. Because of this, she thinks that every time she feels something it means she's pregnant. Or not pregnant. Yeah, I know that makes no sense, but that's kind of the point here.

Depending on the particular day and/or what mood she was in, Julie was ecstatic about feeling that she was really, really pregnant (with twins, even!), or she was crying inconsolably about how she was as barren as the Sahara and she would never have kids. Be prepared for a constant kind of "worst-case scenario theater," where the question "Well, what if . . . ?" is then followed by the most horrible, depressing possibility. "Well, what if we do have twins and one is deformed?" "Well what if we have a baby and I don't love it?" "Well, what if we can't ever have children and one day you leave me for Cameron Diaz when the two of you reach for the same box of Frosted Flakes at the supermarket?" Oh yeah, it's like this, and these are some of the more *lighthearted* concerns. The closer it gets to pregnancy test time the delusions seem to get a whole lot weirder and more paranoid. I'm talking situations involving ghosts, flying squirrels, and former secretary of state Henry Kissinger—that kind of weird.

As the only one not on powerful artificial hormones in our relationship at the time, I tried my hardest to keep Julie on an even keel, telling her that no matter what happened, everything would be alright, if worse truly came to worst we could always try again, the sun'll come up tomorrow—you know, all that placating crap. So what if I didn't believe a single word that came out of my mouth? Didn't matter. This wasn't just about me.

Remember that throughout all of this, you two are a team. And even teammates sometimes need to be reminded that everyone's working for the same goal. Sometimes it can be as simple as telling her you realize that even though it isn't your ass that resembles a dartboard hanging on the wall of an Irish pub, that doesn't mean you aren't feeling the same kinds of anxiety, nervousness, and pain about what's happening that she is.

TESTING, ONE, TWO—WHEE!!!

You and your wife have suffered through weeks, maybe even months, of what can only favorably be compared to hell. The two of you have endured countless doctor visits and drugs and needles and yelling and screaming and fêng shui and throwing spaghetti around the living room (maybe that last one was just us, but I didn't want to leave it out, just in case).

Now comes the moment of truth: the pregnancy test—probably the most important test you'll ever take in your life (yes, that includes the SAT, your driver's test, and meeting your wife's crazy family for the first time). This is also known as the beta test. Why? I have my own theory: If you were a doctor, would you rather say to your patients, "Okay, let's give your wife the blood test that tells whether or not she's pregnant," or instead flash them a serious "doctor look" and state authoritatively, "It's now time to administer . . . the beta test!" I think that second one just sort of *pops*, doesn't it?

The less-exciting truth is that there just happen to be two different levels of hCG—alpha and beta—and the beta levels are evaluated to determine whether you're pregnant or not. Just accept that's what it's called and don't niggle over details. It's beneath you.

Speaking of things being beneath you, if you're overtly emotional, then you're in luck. This happens to be one of the few times in your life you can outwardly show you're nervous without being penalized for having a penis (which I guess would technically be considered "penile-izing").

When Julie and I were going through IVF, I began to notice kind of a weird thing happening: Most of the time our wives really yearn for us to be the strong "manly men of legend" for them—you know, watching football, fixing furniture, killing spiders, etc. On the other hand, if—at least in cases like this—we don't show *enough* emotion, they start to wonder whether we're monstrous sociopaths who keep our feelings bottled up and pushed deep, deep down in our guts until one day we have a complete psychotic break and drive out to the bad part of town to get into fights with bums who really haven't done anything wrong except remind us of our fathers. Maybe not quite that extreme, but they do want to see a little emotion on our parts every now and then, particularly in special cases like this.

Remember that while Mr. Spock has legions of devoted nerd fan boys giving him love by flashing Vulcan hand signs, it was Captain Kirk who got all those hot green space women—and I ask you, is there *anyone* who can emote like William Shatner? I answer with an emphatic "No!" Now, is there a lesson we can take away from all this? On reflection . . . nah, probably not. (But on the upside, I did just win a bet with a friend who said there was *no way* I could slip at least one good *Star Trek* reference somewhere into this book.)

Okay, getting back to business: You're *technically* supposed to go to your doctor and take the blood test anywhere from ten days to two weeks after implantation, at which point the lab analyzes your wife's blood for the telltale beta hCG levels to determine if she's pregnant or not. If you're curious, hCG levels are measured in *milli-international units per milliliter* (mIU/ml)—pretty much the metric system on steroids. Your doctor is looking for an hCG level of somewhere between 5 and 50 mIU/ml; less than 5 mIU/ml is considered negative, while more than 25 mIU/ml is a pretty good indicator that she's pregnant. An especially high number could even signify twins!

You may have noticed that I said "*technically.*" I use that term because I've yet to meet or hear of any IVF couple who actually *waited* for the official blood test before doing a crapload of tests all on their own. Think back to when you were a kid and you couldn't wait for Christmas morning, so instead you went sneaking around the house, searching for where Mom and Dad hid the presents. To be honest, the soon-to-be-pregnant are not a patient bunch; you can't even finish a decent game of Monopoly with them.

But there's a reason you need to wait: Doctors don't arbitrarily pick a date and think, "Yeah, I guess I could tell them tomorrow, but it'd be a lot more fun to screw with their heads." After all, they're not sadists. Well, sure, *some* of them are, but you can usually tell who they are by the copious amounts of studded leather in the exam rooms, and how instead of a gown they have you in assless chaps. By the way, did I mention I live in Los Angeles?

The reason they have you wait the length of time that they do is because they know two weeks is about the average time it takes for those delicate hCG hormone levels to rise just enough in your wife's bloodstream for the lab to be able to get an accurate reading utilizing their complex equipment, including state-of-the-art computers, digital scanners, and precisely calibrated medical centrifuges.

Still, your wife, being the patient woman that she is, will probably run out to the local Walgreens a week early and buy up a shitload of pregnancy pee sticks at three boxes for fifteen bucks. Makes perfect sense, right?

Doctors try to dissuade overeager IVF-ers from testing too soon, mostly because, while the store-bought tests may work just fine, there's always that chance of the false positive or false negative. Either way, it has the potential to screw with your mind, and stress is the last thing you want at this point in the game.

THE CALL OF THE CHILD?

Turnaround time is pretty fast on the beta test. Your wife takes it first thing in the morning, and the two of you get the call anywhere between one and three that afternoon. Again, I say "the two of you," because you're pretty much gonna be taking the day off of work, my friend. I mean seriously, what? Like you're actually going to be sitting in your office and saying to your assistant, "Say, Marcy, if my wife calls do me a favor and put her through—today we're finding out after months of physical and emotional pain and turmoil whether we're pregnant or if we're going to be shattered and forced to reevaluate our goals for parenthood once again. Oh, and can you also get me the latest cost analysis on the Phillips project? Thanks." Nope, you're cashing in a personal day, bub. If it makes you feel any better, go ahead and rationalize it as a test: If your office can't run without you for a day, then chances are the place is going to slide into the crapper pretty soon anyway. Hey, better to find out *before* the kid needs braces, right?

Okay, obviously, when the call comes in, you'll have two possible scenarios:

1. Scenario one: It's positive!

Congratulations! It's been a long time coming, and from this point on, you're going to be feeling a lot of things at once: ecstasy, confusion, nervousness.

You'll have to go back into the doctor's office every couple of days to make sure the beta levels are rising (they should be doubling every couple of days), and after a few weeks, you get to say, "Goodbye, fertility doctor" and "Hello, ob-gyn!" That part I can't help you with, but don't worry. Your wife already has one picked out. Really. She does. Ask her.

2. Scenario two: It's negative.

I'm sorry. Really, I am. It's one thing to have an earlier phase of the protocol fail, but to get as far as you
have and find out there is no finish line to cross . . .
that's just awful. You're going to have some feelings here as well, except they're going to be pretty
damn negative ones. You're also going to have to be
the rock your wife can cling to during this time.
Again, sexist sounding as it may be, you as the man
have a very specific role here, and she's going to
need you to be there for her.

What you shouldn't do, however, is give up hope. Recon-
nect with your doctor; get him to debrief you on the whole
protocol. Talk to him about what he thinks might have gone
wrong and where it might have happened. It's been said that
IVF is just as much an art as it is a science. Each IVF cycle is
a learning experience, each one guiding the doctor closer
and closer to the chemistry equation that will finally result
in your pregnancy.

Of course, if you choose not to go the IVF road again,
there are still a lot of ways you and your beloved can become parents—in most cases ways you never even thought of.
I'll go into more detail about these later, but know that in this
crazy, wacky scientific world of the future, if you really, really want a child, in most cases you can have one. It's just
going to take a *lot* of work.

SEVEN

Sperm-a-Lot

So it all comes down to this. You're in "The Room," a plastic cup in one hand, an erotic (yet tasteful) men's magazine in the other. On the other side of the door, a whole room full of highly trained medical professionals (oh, and your wife too), all of them just . . . *waiting*. And all you can think is "How the hell did I get here?"

This is the scene most people think of when they think IVF. Well, it's the part most men think of, anyway. I say that because it was the part I thought of.

AND KNOWING IS HALF THE BATTLE!

During one of our first office visits, when my wife and I quizzed our doctor about what the actual fertilization procedure would entail, he explained my wife's part in explicit detail: She would be put under a twilight anesthesia and her oocytes would be collected by ultrasound-guided follicle aspiration, etc. She continually nodded as, God bless her, she understood every bit of what he was saying.

I nodded too, but only because I didn't want to look stupid. "Aspirated follicles?" I asked myself. "What the hell does her hair have to do with making a baby?" And yet still I nodded, because, well, I am a man, and I know everything—even the stuff I don't know. (Oh, by the way, my lack of that particular little tidbit of knowledge would come back and bite me in the butt later. But I digress.)

One thing I did realize, though, is that no one really talked to me about what my part in this little baby-making venture would be. Even reading through the library of books my wife had bought didn't help. I barely rated a mention. But that was okay, since I kind of pieced together an idea . . .

At some point, I would be whisked off to a private room—a softly lit, comfortable hidden enclave stocked with all forms of male stimulation. And eventually, after plenty of . . . alone time, I would discreetly place my full sample cup into some kind of vacuum tube where it would be deposited directly into the doctor's sure and steady hand. And then—the miracle of conception!

Ah, I do lead a rich and creative fantasy life. The reality is somewhat more, well, *real*.

FEELS LIKE THE FIRST TIME

I have no idea what kind of guy you are. You may be a Fortune 500 executive, with the power to hire and fire thousands at the slightest whim. You may be the finest rodeo rider in all of South Texas, with every bull in the state quaking at the mere sound of your spurs. You may even be a navy test pilot, flying a top secret experimental Q–14 Suborbital Stealth Strike Fighter. (NOTE TO THE PENTAGON: I just totally made that name up. If, however, there is indeed some top secret aircraft buzzing around with that name, I humbly ask that you not have me killed. I know nothing.) You may be the manliest of men, but nothing will prepare you for the time when you must submit your sperm for judgment.

Think back to your first time. You know what I mean. Remember how nervous you were? Remember how unsure you felt? "What if I don't stack up?" "What if I suck?" "What if right in the middle I start crying—?" Alright, maybe I opened up a little too much with that one. In any case, that same combination of nerves, trepidation, and all-out fear is what you should expect to feel your first time in The Room.

I hear what you're asking. "First time? Whoa, whoa, wait a minute—I thought all I have to do is come and go!" Well, yes and no.

Yes, as in "Yes, I know that's what you thought," and no, as in "No, you couldn't be more wrong."

'CAUSE I'M NOT . . . I'M NOT
THAT STRONG A SWIMMER

Before your doctor can help you figure out which fertility treatment might be best for you, several aspects of your semen and sperm must be analyzed and reviewed. Chief among these are concentration, volume, motility, and morphology. Let's take a look at them, shall we?

Concentration is exactly what it sounds like: the amount of sperm present per milliliter of semen. (Measurement of semen is done metrically, just like in fine cooking. Uh, I probably shouldn't have written those two things into the same sentence. Sorry.) According to the World Health Organization (WHO), the ideal number is over 20 million per milliliter.[e] Anything less is known as *oligospermia*, which is more or less a fancy way of saying, "Your six-shooter's firing blanks there, pardner!"

If you are diagnosed with a low sperm count, don't beat yourself up. In today's wacky, modern, go-go world, lots of possible behavioral and environmental causes could be to blame, including:

- Drug use (now really, was it worth it just to see if Pink Floyd's *The Wall* synched up with *The Wizard of Oz*?).

- Excessive smoking (hey, at least you looked cool).

- High fevers.

- Hot tubs, saunas (they're so seventies anyway).

- Chemotherapies.

- Radiation exposure (this would explain why there weren't any little Incredible Hulk-lings stomping around the Banner household).

Of course, there's also the very real possibility that it's all just genetics, which means it's purely bad cosmic luck that your army's going off to war a few divisions short. Even if that is the case, buck up! As we learned earlier, when it comes to IVF you may need only one, lonely little sperm!

Volume is, well, volume. How much you can come up with, so to speak. Somewhere between one and six and a half milliliters of semen is considered to be within the "normal range." If you're producing less than that, even though it's not exactly ideal, there are still fertility methods that can work for you. If you're producing more? Well, hats off to you, my friend! (As an added bonus, there might even be a future for you in certain videos made in the San Fernando Valley.)

The next important measurement is *motility*. Basically, this is the movement of the sperm. Again, going by the WHO guidelines, the standard for what they consider a "motility norm" is 50 percent of observed sperm showing some kind of forward movement. So with the aforementioned 20 million sperm, 10 million of them have to be headed in the right direction for your boys to be considered "normal."

Oddly enough, the whole "more is always better" theory doesn't necessarily apply to a good motility measurement, because even if a man has plenty of volume (say, a concentration of over 20 million sperm per milliliter), he still needs at least 50 percent with good motility in order to have what's considered "decent-quality sperm." Conversely, a man with much less concentration may actually have a higher motility percentage, and thus his sperm may be even better quality than those of Mr. "I've got 20 million and you don't."

Let's put it another way: A top-of-the-line Ferrari sitting in your driveway may look like a sweet dream ride, but if you don't have an engine under the hood, all you've got is a quarter-million-dollar gas can.

The final important measurement is *morphology*—and no, it has nothing to do with brightly colored Power Rangers. It relates to the shape of your sperm, and how well they conform to what is considered a "normal, good-looking sperm." Ideally, 14–30 percent of your sperm should fall into this category. The rest of them can look like Joe Pesci for all you care.

Male fertility problems could be indicated by low scores in any, or all, of these measurements. In my case, it was the big trifecta of volume, motility, and morphology. To use a sports analogy, you know how during the relay swimming events in the Summer Olympics the camera almost always seems to follow the American and Australian swimmers in the middle lanes—you know, the really good-looking guys and girls who seem to break all of the world records?

Well, if we think of those folks as "ideal sperm," then my sperm would be the out-of-shape guy from Turkmenistan who's just sort of half assing a dog-paddle in lane eight. Believe me, it wasn't exactly the news my wife and I were hoping for, but it was good to know, because now we had a clear picture of what we were dealing with, and what our options were.

IT'S ABOUT TIME

Okay, now that you know what it is the doctor will be looking for, the big question is "How are they going to get it from me?" Well, I'm sure you can figure out "how" they intend to get it from you, but the *how* of the how can be an ordeal in itself. This isn't any ordinary run-of-the-mill session with yourself. ("Oh, um, I was in the shower an extra, extra long time 'cause I wanted my hair really, really clean.") No sir. This is the most organized self-love session of your life.

First there's an abstinence period, usually two to seven days. This allows your reserves to build up, and gives the lab a decent sample to work with. You and I both know that married or not, there've been times you've gone way longer than that. You'll live.

Now, despite the fact that the clinic may sometimes tell you that you can collect your sample at home and bring it in, that's generally inadvisable. For one thing, the sample must be at the doctor's office within sixty to ninety minutes of collection, due to the chemical changes the semen undergoes. It's vitally important for the sperm to be "washed out" or separated from the rest of the seminal fluid as soon as possible, and most labs need their samples first thing in the morning. If you live in or near a major city, early in the morning means you're not getting anywhere within sixty to ninety minutes.

"Eh," you say dismissively, "I can make it. I'll just speed. No problem." Okay, but you're taking a big risk. The last thing you want is to be pulled over by the police while carrying a container of your own man-gravy in your lap. Not only will you miss your drop-off-time window, but once you've explained to the officer exactly what it is sloshing around in that cup between your legs, well, unless he's the cop from the Village People, your answer isn't exactly going to endear you to him. So, just decide now to deposit directly at the clinic. It's a good choice. Trust me.

Now, you'll need to make an appointment at the fertility clinic. Yes, you heard me correctly: You have to phone ahead for a masturbation. As I mentioned before, these appointments are almost always scheduled for the early, early morning. The reason for this is that the lab techs need time to run all of the tests on the samples, as well as prepare the sperm for any fertilization procedures scheduled for that day. It's usually a full docket, so the best advice is to get there early.

Alright, so you're showered and shaved (your face, I mean—you know, unless you're into that kind of thing) and you've arrived at the clinic, ready to do what you have to do. Allow me to take you through your visit, step by step:

JUST CHECKING IN

Let's face it. No matter how secure you are as a man, it's not the easiest thing in the world to walk into a fertility clinic. And this is due in no small part to the fact that you're probably going to be signing in with a receptionist who will almost invariably be a young, cute blonde, to whom you will have to mutter, "I'm here for the lab." (Of course, in your mind it sounds like, "Hey, I'm going to watch some porn and pleasure myself for a while! Do you validate?")

Look, don't worry about it, because—guess what?—she already knows why you're there. I mean, come on, she works at a fertility clinic for God's sake! It's not like random guys are dropping by just for the coffee.

At this point she will direct you toward the lab. Now this is where it really, really pays to get there early. I mean "as soon as they open" early. If you're the first one there, great! Move right on to the next step. If you're not, then you've got a little bit of a wait in store, as those men who didn't stop off for that grande latte are going to get in ahead of you.

THE WAITING IS THE HARDEST PART

For men, the waiting room of a fertility clinic can be a little ominous, a little foreboding. Hell, it can be just plain weird. If you walk into the waiting room and see a woman sitting there all by herself, there are many possibilities as to what her story is: Maybe she's part of a married couple and the man couldn't make it to the appointment that day. Perhaps she's trying to become a single mother. She could be one-half of a lesbian couple. It's difficult to say.

When you see a man sitting alone in a fertility clinic waiting room, there's only one reason he's there. You know it. He knows it. Even the guy delivering bottled water to the office knows it. Now, if you happen to be one of the thirty-or-so men in the western hemisphere who didn't have their egos crushed like Hummel figurines in an elephant stampede at some point in their lives (probably high school—no, definitely high school) and you're just bristling with poise and exuding self-confidence, this won't be a problem for you. Good for you. Go to hell.

For the rest of us guys, this can be rather embarrassing. Furtive eye movements, averted glances, and squirming in seats are not uncommon behaviors. (It also doesn't help that these waiting rooms are invariably stocked with magazines like *Us Weekly*, *People*, and *Cosmo*. Look, it's not like we're asking for *Bass Fishing Monthly* or *Soldier of Fortune*, but come on!)

Another thing that makes it worse than it probably should be is that we're all sizing one another up, hoping against hope that we're not going in after the skeezy-looking guy with the torn sweatpants and the long greasy hair poking out from underneath the knit cap he's wearing in eighty-degree weather. Ugh.

And then, finally, you're summoned. You take a deep breath and get up—again, careful not to make eye contact with anyone—and walk off into the great unknown that is The Room.

AN EMPTY ROOM,
A PLASTIC CUP, AND THOU

Okay, you've finally arrived. This is where the magic happens. Now remember when I described the wonderful, Nirvana-like place where a man can relax and let it all hang out? Bullshit. Total crap. Doesn't exist. It may vary from place to place, but at my clinic, I found myself standing outside of a small 6 x 7 foot exam room, which was lit by bright medical fluorescent bulbs and furnished with a paper sheet–covered chair in the middle of the floor and a 12" TV/DVD combo on the sink. Wow. Talk about a letdown. Now I know how my wife feels every Valentine's Day.

The lab tech then handed me a specimen cup and I was told to "be sure to lock the door," and that was it. Suddenly it was just me and my . . . well, *me*.

Now, I'm going to stop here and, in the spirit of the Boy Scouts' motto "Be prepared," pass along a few things I had to learn for myself. It actually took a few times at bat to figure them out, but now I gladly pass them on to you. So, I present a little breakdown of what to expect, and what not to expect on your big day.

1. Prepare to chafe—badly.

Unfortunately, the multitudes of lubricants, both natural and industrial, which have provided us men with so much blisterless joy over the years, may contaminate the sample, as they are quite nonconducive to the purity of the semen the lab wishes to obtain. Translation: You're doing it dry. Ouch.

2. Consider bringing your own material.

While the fertility clinics do help you out by providing you with a few stimuli, they aren't necessarily known for their taste in porn. Their collection is mostly made up of some back issues of Playboy and a few videos straight out of the bargain bin at the local adult emporium. Seriously, the ones I saw still had the $5.00 markdown stickers, and as we all know, you can't get decent porn for less than $14.95.

Now, the more prudish of you may think it untoward that this beautiful, precious little life you're striving to bring into the world basically started with you sitting all alone watching a threesome involving two Asian cheerleaders. But just remember, it's all for the greater good. Besides, this is one time your wife doesn't mind you watching it, so take advantage. Oh, and while we're on the subject of the videos . . .

3. Make sure you take your video out before you leave!

This is more of a common courtesy thing than anything else. Think of it as an adult "Be kind, rewind" policy. I mean, if you were to sit down and press the eject button and out pops a disc full of some weird, creepy eastern European midget porn (just an example of course . . .), that's going to make something that's already difficult a lot more difficult-er. Or something like that.

In a similar vein, do not steal the videos from the office. You've already spent at least a few thousand on the fertility treatments. Be a sport and go buy your own smut.

4. Write your name on the cup before you use it.

In general, it's always a good idea. And last, but certainly not least . . .

5. You don't have to fill the whole cup!

Remember, the average man has an ejaculation of somewhere between one and six and a half milliliters. The cup they give you to use holds about two ounces. If you actually did try to fill the whole thing, you'd be dead from dehydration and your boy would be whittled down into a Slim Jim before you got anywhere close. Don't try to be a hero. It's not worth it.

PLEASE MAKE SURE
YOU SHOW ALL YOUR WORK

At last! You've done it! You're the proud holder of a cup with some semen in it. Good for you. Last part is to drop it off with the lab tech. It's not like when you give a urine sample and you can just leave it in the restroom, or when they tell you to put it in that lazy susan thingy mounted in the wall that makes the cup disappear like one of those trick haunted-house bookcases on *Scooby Doo*.

Nope, you actually have to walk that bad boy over to the lab tech. "I can't do that!" you say. "Walking around with a cup of my own sperm in my hand? What am I, a Sigma Chi?" (Okay, okay, that was cheap. Everyone knows it's the Sig Eps who do that.) But you know what? Once again, no one there cares.

You have to remember that this sort of thing is their stock-in-trade. If anything, you should be happy. You should be proud. You've done what few men would have the guts, the determination to do. You've taken a major step toward your ultimate goal of creating a child—of forming a family. So go forth and hold your head high, walk right up to the lab tech, put your sample cup down on the counter, and proclaim in a loud voice, "I am a man, and by God, this is my semen! Do you validate?"

EIGHT

Real Men Don't Cry
(However, They Do
Sometimes
Quietly Sob into
Their Pillows)

We all know that men and women are, at the core of it, different in the ways they look at life: In ancient tribal societies, women were gatherers and men were hunters. In today's society, women are the shoppers and men are the mill-around-the-shoe-departments-while-she's-trying-on-things-ers. There's even that hoary old axiom that women are very emotional and men are strictly logical.

We men have been conditioned from birth not to be overly emotional. We're told all through our childhood to "suck it up," "play through the pain," "walk it off," "stop doing that or you'll go blind." Okay, the last one doesn't really apply, but I do vividly remember being told that several times.

Even today, though we're living in a world where a guy can be called a "metrosexual" and it isn't considered a put-down, where males get liposuction and calf implants instead of (gasp!) *actually working out*, and where a guy like Matt Damon is passed off as an action hero, we men have certain expectations. We're expected to open the doors for women, we're expected to be the breadwinners in our families, and we're not supposed to show emotions like sadness or depression or guilt.

Unfortunately for so many of us in the world of fertility treatments, we know that not only are those feelings real, but they tend to hang out and rattle around our heads 24/7 like those crappy beaded curtains in the back of a customized 1970s van. What you have to do is learn how to deal with what you're feeling, and how not to let it ruin what should be the most important time in your and your wife's lives.

"Oh, crap," I hear you saying. "This is where the book is gonna get all mushy and touchy-feely and *Oprah* on me." Please, after all we've been through in here, would I do that to you? What I do want to do is reassure you that anything and everything you're feeling is really common, and that you're not some sort of failure just because things aren't going "the way they should." Because if there's one thing you can learn from fertility treatments, it's that nothing goes the way it should.

DID YOU TRY WHACKING IT A COUPLE OF TIMES?

Now traditionally, when a couple experiences problems having children, you'd think it must be the woman, right? "After all," the common logic goes, "she's the one actually having the kid, so there must be something going on inside of her." Ah, but you, being the smart man-about-town that you are (plus having read the first few chapters of this book), also know that a lot can go wrong with a guy's plumbing.

I'm a prime example: When we went to see a fertility specialist for some testing, it turned out that the baby-making problem wasn't Julie. It was yours truly. My sperm was, to put it mildly, poor grade. How poor of a grade was it? If it was one of my students and it tested like that, I would have arranged a conference with its parents and suggested that it be held back a year—hell, maybe two, just to play it safe. That's how poor a grade it was.

Sure, I can joke about it now, but when the doctor handed me the lab report—the numbers on my sperm count reading lower than the ratings on a PBS documentary on wildebeest migrations—yeah, it was kind of a big deal. I tried to keep it together. Being a man, I was supposed to be strong, right? Outwardly, I was all smiles and sunshine: "Okay, well, at least now we know what the problem is, so let's just go ahead and see what we can do about it." Ah, but inside . . . inside, I was crushed. Really, truly devastated. More than that, I was embarrassed. I mean, what kind of man was I if I couldn't even get my wife pregnant?

BUT THINK OF ALL
YOU'LL SAVE ON CONDOMS!

At the risk of sounding crude, let me start out this section saying that throughout my premarried dating life, I was always proud that I never once accidentally got a girl pregnant. I doubt they give out Boy Scout patches for it (wow, I hope they don't!) but if they did, I would definitely have earned mine. All around me were friends telling horror stories about their own "mistakes," but not me! My record was spotless.

And now, there in the fertility doctor's office, I found out why. Damn. You have to admit, there's kind of a sick irony in it: The very thing that let me dodge bullets like Wyatt Earp walking the creek in *Tombstone* before was now standing in the way of my having a family.

What made me feel worse was the fact that this was the one thing I figured I didn't need to worry about. It seems simple enough: I'm a man; men get their wives pregnant and have babies. But then it turned out I couldn't get my wife pregnant, at least not naturally, so what did that say about my manhood?

LET'S TALK ABOUT OUR FEELINGS— BUT WAIT TILL HALFTIME, OKAY?

As men, that seems to be a suggestion no one ever offers us. When women find out one of their friends is having trouble conceiving, everyone gets together and comforts her, and they talk it over and sip wine and then get silly and dance around the living room table to a classic song from the sixties (granted, I kind of sussed that out from watching movies on Lifetime, Oxygen, and We).

Unfortunately, we guys don't have that kind of support system. Sure, we like Motown and the British invasion bands as much as any woman, but it's just not in our nature to sit around talking—and certainly not about anything like infertility or our feelings about it. I mean, what are we supposed to say? "Y'know, Mike, this whole situation just makes me feel like . . . well, like less of a man." The answer we'd probably hear would be a simple "Eh, just suck it up," followed by a request to pass the blue cheese dip for the wings.

No, in a case like this, the first link in your support system needs to be your wife. You'd be there for her if it turned out she were the one having the problem, right? Of course you would. Like I've said before, you two are a team, a united front against all obstacles—even the ones blocking your seminal vesicles. You should want to talk to her about this, and ideally, she should want to listen.

Now I know that no man wants to look weak in front of his woman; how many of us still remember that furniture-moving escapade when she asked us, "Are you sure that isn't too heavy?" as we grinned through the massive "insta-hernia" we got attempting to move a 500-pound sectional across the room all by ourselves? Opening yourself up emotionally to anyone, especially your wife, can be very difficult. Admitting you're feeling bad about a perceived weakness is a big step, but if you've reached this point, nothing can be gained by holding back.

Emotions can't be denied. They can be channeled, repressed, dammed up—any other metaphors you'd like to use—but they're gonna come out. If you're having a bad day at work, you're going to take it out on someone, whether it's your assistant, your co-worker, or the barista who accidentally gives you half caf instead of decaf. And that's just work. If you have a game changer like infertility suddenly appear, do you really think you can deny the bad feelings it's going to stir up? Meditate all you want, my friend, but every time you look at one of your friends' kids, you're going to think to yourself, "Why the hell can't I have one of those? God, I suck."

If you can't talk to your wife, then you need to talk to someone. Find a therapist who deals with infertility issues. I kid you not; they're out there. There're enough of us around that it is actually a lucrative specialty. Talking with one, either by yourself or as a couple, can help you come to grips with what you're going through, which in turn makes it easier to move on to the next step (the fertility treatment).

HEY, DON'T LOOK AT ME!

Now if it happens to be your wife who has the fertility problem, that can engender a whole other set of negative feelings. Only this time it's not *self*-loathing you need to worry about.

Men are biologically wired to "procreate," but women are hardwired to be "mommies." Deny it they might, but it's a fact of life. There's a difference between the sexes. According to a recent study cited in the *American Journal of Play* (yes, it's a real thing!) even if you deny little boys access to toy guns, they'll pick up sticks and start to go "Bang, bang!" Conversely, if there are no dolls around to play with, little girls will cradle bundles of sticks and pretend they are babies.[f]

If and when a woman learns she is infertile, or even has fertility problems, this is a monstrous blow to her. Her primary biological purpose in life is threatened, and she's not going to take it well at all. Remember when I just said how you two need to work as a united front? This is where you need to be there for her. And it won't be easy, for a number of reasons.

Think about when you got married, and you found out there was a very good reason she always seemed to make that rockin' chicken marsala for you: It's all she knew how to make. Now in this day and age, a woman who doesn't spend her whole life in the kitchen isn't that big of a surprise. After all, that's why God created take-out. Anyway, this probably didn't equate to a major deal breaker in your mind.

Okay, now consider this scenario: You're about to get married, and you suddenly learn your betrothed can't have children, or at least is going to have a lot of trouble conceiving. Do you shrug it off? If you're a man who wants a family, probably not. There's a reason for that. Women are expected to have babies, the same way men are expected to kill spiders. (Actually, I try to save them and take them outside. I'd expect the same courtesy if and when I ever run into a giant mutated arachnid one day. I'm a firm believer in karma.) If you take away a woman's ability to have a child, of course something precious has been stolen. And it's not just something that was stolen from *her*; this also now affects you too. Any plans you may have had of being a daddy have suddenly disappeared. It means you're losing the chance to toss the ball around the backyard with Bud, and you won't be playing "mean Dad" and scaring some respectability into Kitten's prom date. That's some very real and heavy stuff to find yourself dealing with. So where do you go from here?

SORRY, MR. FIX IT—YOU CAN'T FIX IT

How many times have you been in a situation when your wife comes to you with a problem, goes off on a ten-minute rant, and then, at the end, when you offer up a flawlessly thought out, perfectly executed solution to the problem, she gets angry, saying, "I don't want your advice! I was just venting!"

This mindset is obviously completely whacked-out to us men. As the timeless philosophers from Devo put it oh so well, "When a problem comes along, you must whip it." As I've mentioned earlier, men, by nature, are problem solvers. Can't hunt a wooly mammoth by yourself? Get a group of friends together. That drill cord isn't long enough? String together a whole bunch of extension cords. TV's not working? Smack it around until the newscaster's face looks a slightly less disturbing shade of blue. This is who we are, and this is what we do. When your wife comes to you with a problem, your first inclination is to solve the problem, because as the great man-logic equation dictates: problem + solution = no more problem. Hey, it's our system, and it works.

Now along comes infertility to throw a major kink into that system, a male brain scrambler, the tic-tac-toe game to the Wargames computer that is the male mind (and if you get that reference, you *rock*!). You want to come up with a fix, but you can't. This "does not compute" situation can drive a huge wedge into a marriage, as emotions like guilt and anger, left unaddressed, can eat away at your relationship.

MIND YOUR OWN BEESWAX!

Another issue you're going to have to deal with is the pressure of other people knowing what you're going through. Fertility treatments are not something you can keep to yourself, like your video rental record during your twenties. Nope, get ready for the questions, because everyone around you is going to know about it.

It's impossible to keep it a secret. Your wife is going to tell her friends, who will tell their friends. Of course you're going to have to let your family know and then they'll tell people. It's like a damn shampoo commercial. Don't get me wrong, they'll be supportive; hell, they may even be too supportive. They'll always be asking: "How's it going?" Giving you advice: "Just relax, it'll happen!" Offering stories: "I knew this couple, they tried and tried, and then, one day, they had triplets! I know that'll happen to you!" And quasi counseling: "You must feel awful, huh?" Really insightful stuff there.

This is where you need to grow a really thick skin. There's nothing you can do about the prying eyes, and yes, you could yell at them and tell them to back off, that they have no idea what they're talking about, that they need to go through what you've gone through before they can give opinions. But that would be mean. You're not mean. Instead, just thank them politely, and change the subject. After a few times, they'll take the hint. And if they don't, just stab them in the eye with a shrimp fork. Either way you won't be talking about fertility treatments anymore, right?

UNLESS YOU SEE A BURNING BUSH TOO, IT'S NOT GOD

The last emotional hurdle usually comes when an infertility treatment fails to work. And it does—again, and again. You're going to start feeling like the universe is against you, that

God himself doesn't want you to procreate. Unless you're dead set on giving birth to the Antichrist, I'm going to guarantee you that God has no personal stake in stopping you from conceiving. This is all on mankind.

Again, fertility treatments are an art just as much as they are a science. Each time, the doctors adjust their treatments according to what they saw happen the previous time. The problem is that unless your name happens to be Bob Citibank, you're eventually going to run out of money for these treatments. More than that, you're going to run out of hope.

Fertility treatments are long and trying ordeals. Your wife has to go through hell, both her body and her emotions run ragged by the protocols. You have to be there for her, and at the same time deal with your life too. This can go on for months. The goodness in this is that when she finally gets pregnant, she's going to be able to deal with symptoms that could knock a mere mortal woman out, because she's basically already been through a kind of twisted hardcore pregnancy SEAL training boot camp with all this crap. The bad side is that if it fails, she's headed for a crash faster than a rich kid in a Porsche.

As I said, you might want to look into fertility counseling to help you—to help you both. No one should have to deal with all of these pressures on his own, especially if you have no idea what to expect or how to handle them (which kind of covers . . . oh, everyone). Don't feel too manly to look for help. It'll save you both a lot of heartache in the future.

Fertility treatments are not for the emotionally devoid. You and your wife will need to talk to one another, to communicate what you're feeling and what you're thinking. Many marriages have been irrevocably damaged because of deep-seated tensions. No matter which fertility treatment you end up choosing, odds are it's going to be a long and arduous process. If you listen to any one thing I have to say here, it's that you shouldn't try to handle things all alone; otherwise you run the risk of eventually ending up exactly that—all alone.

NINE

What a Prick!

*W*hen you mention the word "shots," I think it's pretty fair to say that most people prefer the ones you get at a bar versus the ones you get from a doctor—but if your doctor has a full bar at his office, well, you're golden. (You also probably have the makings of a pretty good malpractice suit too, but you can take that up later with your lawyer.)

Now, before we go on, I need to make sure you know two things: 1) when it comes to many types of infertility treatments, it's gonna be injections-a-poppin' for weeks at a clip for your wife, and 2) hopefully you've come to terms with the fact that *you*, my friend, will be the one administering these shots.

Look, as much as you may hate to admit it, fertility treatments are a team project: Your doctor has his part, your wife has her part, and you have your part, which in this case happens to be giving your wife these shots, so nut up and do what a man's gotta do. Trust me, on the fateful day when you'll be called to active duty to change your baby's neurotoxin-laden diapers after his or her first butternut-squash-and-apples puree, you'll think back on this as one of your *fonder* memories.

YOU WANT TO PUT WHAT WHERE?

Whichever fertility treatment you eventually decide to try, there's going to be some kind of medication involved. Whether it's Clomid or Lupron or Follistim or even good ol' Mr. Progesterone, it will seem as if your wife is always taking something to boost this or regulate that. You may ask why she can't just take a pill. I mean, wouldn't that be a whole lot easier? Just gulp down a handful of hGC in the morning, some more in the afternoon, and then a sensible meal for dinner. Please, you're smarter than that! Think about what happens when you take an aspirin. You've seen those commercials with the cutout side view of the person after he swallows the pill: It takes a trip down his throat, hits his tummy, and then gets sent out all over his body to do its job.

That's *not* what we want here. With a few exceptions, fertility meds need to be site specific, so injections are the best way to get what we want where we want it. The question is where are these injectables injected? We're used to shots in our arms, oh, sure, maybe even in our butts. But for this, you're going to need to amp things up and take it one step beyond: These shots go right into her *stomach*. More specifically, you'll be giving your wife most of these injections in that subcutaneous layer of fat at the bottom of her belly.

Just to warn you, your wife is going to hate you for this on two counts: first, for the pain you will be causing her, and second, for the nightly reminder that she does, in fact, have a layer of fat at the bottom of her belly.

AND YOU THOUGHT STICKING NEEDLES
IN FRUIT WAS ONLY FOR HALLOWEEN?

When the actual time comes for the injections, you will visit your doctor and he (or a nurse), will take you and your wife into his office with the idea of showing you how to give the shots. Now remember, these injections will have to be given every day for a couple of weeks. It doesn't sound like a lot, but at three injections per day, it adds up fast. By the time you're done, your sharps container (the little red plastic pail with a safety top where you discard your old needles) will look like a heroin junkie's lunchbox.

I don't think I'm spilling any secrets when I say that men have a tendency to be cavalier about just about anything dangerous, even if we're scared just as shitless as everyone else. Case in point: When Julie and I went in for the lesson on the injectables, she was (rightfully) nervous. Me? I was skipping around, making jokes, playing with the little plastic wombs in the doctor's office and making them talk—real jerk stuff. When the nurse showed me the hypodermic needles I'd be using, I completely freaked out—inside. Outside, I picked it up, pretended to play darts with it, started chasing Julie around the room like Norman Bates in *Psycho*, and generally acted like a complete ass to cover up my insecurity. It's okay to do that. They're used to "guy behavior" there. After all, they're the ones with a whole room full of porn just for us, remember?

Now depending on what your doctor is into, they'll have

you practice on something besides your wife the first time. Some doctors use a ball with a neoprene covering that has the same feel and resistance as human skin, while some go old-school and just make you stick the needle into an orange. Either way, unless you have some deep-seated fetish I don't even want to know about, it's going to feel weird that first time. Don't worry if you think you're doing it wrong; the nurse will be watching closely to make sure you do it right, and your wife will be looking even more closely because she doesn't trust you and thinks you're going to kill her.

Be prepared for your wife to be . . . a tad unsure about your skills here. In my case, as every step was explained and demonstrated to me, Julie would ask, "Did you see that? Did you see how she did it? Do you need her to show you again? Maybe she should show you again. Did you bring your glasses?" Me: "Sweetie, I don't wear glasses." Julie: "Right. Well maybe we should wait until you go to the optometrist and get some glasses!"

Truth be told, she kind of had a right to be nervous. Taking an impartial look back at things, Julie was sitting there on the exam table watching me stab at that practice ball with my needle like I was checking the interior temperature of a roast. What can I say? Up until that point my sole medical experience was limited to a season or two of *ER* and that old Operation game I played when I was a kid—so unless George Clooney came bursting in with a massive head-trauma case or Julie's nose suddenly turned red and *buzzed*, I was pretty much lost.

GREG WOLFE

"JUST RELAX, SWEETIE—
I HAVE NO IDEA WHAT I'M DOING"

Okay, so you're back at home, and the time has come. Your wife has talked to the doctor about her cycle, and everyone has agreed that now's the time to start the protocol. Gulp.

This first injection is really key; it sets the tone for all the injections to come. You screw this one up in a major way, and she'll think you're always going to screw it up. And this includes measuring out the dose, prepping the injection site, giving her the shot, and post-shot procedures. Yes, each of these is critical. Later on, once she's confident in your skills, you can muck around a little bit (we all do . . .), but this first one is key.

What you'll want to do, or at least give the appearance of doing, is take your time. Some of these medications come prepackaged; others you actually have to mix (don't worry, I'll walk you through it). Remember, your wife is allowing you, a guy that can barely make a decent manhattan, to play mad scientist in the bathroom, mixing up and then injecting her with powerful hormones. Yeah, this is a *huge* deal. Think about it: Whom would you trust to give you a shot, aside from your doctor? Your poker buddies? Half the time you have to remind those dummies that a flush beats a straight. She's giving up a lot of control here, so please, humor her neuroses during the first few days.

So, now that the warnings are out of the way, let's take a walk through the series of injections, shall we?

GETTING LOOPY WITH LUPRON

The initial medication for an IVF cycle is going to be Lupron, or something very much like it, which, as you'll remember, is a luteinizing hormone used to stop her from ovulating. Now for you, this is going to be the easiest of the shots. Easiest because:

1. It's the smallest needle and syringe you'll be using.

2. It already comes premixed in its own vial.

Notice I said this will be the easiest for *you*, not for her. For her, this is going to be the most difficult thing she's ever done, even if she's a professional cliff diver. The needle itself is only ¼ inch long. Yeah, I know; that doesn't sound like much, but to your wife, it'll look like a Patriot missile heading right for her midsection. Again, taking your time with the first few shots will help immensely with the next round of injections, which definitely *will* be a pain, for both of you.

So, let's go through it step by step. To begin with, you should have the following:

- the vial of Lupron

- a box of 25 gauge, ¼ inch hypodermic syringes

- rubbing alcohol pads (the prepackaged ones work better than a cotton ball dipped in rubbing alcohol)

- gauze pads

- a copy of *Lethal Weapon (Director's Cut)* on DVD
  (you don't need it for the injections, but it's an
  awesome movie and you really *should* have it)

Okay, now that we're all set, let's do this.

STEP ONE — Clean it Up

So, the first thing you need to do is make sure everything is clean. That means you, your workspace (I mixed all our shots up in the kitchen, so Clorox Clean-up Cleaner with Bleach was my best friend), your equipment—everything.

Start by unwrapping an alcohol pad and wiping off the rubber stopper in the Lupron bottle. This is something you want to get into the habit of doing, because you're going to wipe off every lid of every medication you use, be it cap, stopper, cork, or pull tab. (Just kidding, there are no pull-tab medications—although a good can of Guinness comes awfully close.)

STEP TWO — Load it Up

Alright, so now that we're ready, it's time to load it up:

1. Take the syringe and pull back on the plunger all the way to the amount prescribed by your doctor, usually 1cc.

2. Carefully push the needle through the rubber stopper of the Lupron vial. (IMPORTANT NOTE: Don't bend the needle!)

3. Holding the syringe steady, turn both the syringe and the bottle upside down. Push down on the plunger of the syringe, all the way to the bottom, then release. If you did this right, the syringe will automatically fill up with the correct amount of Lupron.

4. Carefully remove the syringe, then, holding the syringe needle up, push slightly on the plunger, expelling any leftover air, until a drop or two of Lupron shows up at the tip. (NOTE: If you see the liquid shoot across the room like it was launched out of some kind of Nerf water blaster, then you probably pressed a *little* too hard.)

5. Make sure the Lupron vial goes back into the fridge. Don't leave it out. Not only will it ruin the drug, but your wife will find it laying on the counter and rip into you as if you were a Pringles can. Yeah. So remember: Lupron. Fridge. Pringles.

And once that fridge door is closed, *voilà!* You just made yourself up an injection like them fancy doctor types do on the TV. Now recap the needle before you poke yourself in the eye.

STEP THREE — Numb it Up

Now comes the fun part. Like I said, your wife is going to be freaking out at this point. Not only is she like everyone else in the world and scared to death of sharp things coming at her, but in this case it's a sharp thing wielded by a heretofore un-trained amateur who can't even remember to wipe the tooth-paste globs out of the sink each morning.

But this is where you get to show her! This is where you set the tone for every injection to come afterward. Imagine her on the phone with her friends, bragging about your manly, confident demeanor, your amazing technique, your sure, steady hands. Like most things in life, attitude is every-thing here. Even if you're scared shitless—stomach tied up in knots, sweat soaking through your undershirt to the point you feel like you just got off of Splash Mountain—you had better be really good at pretending you're not. Women love to see confidence in a guy, especially in a guy who's just about to stab them in the stomach.

So what do you do? Simple: You fake it. You just keep smiling and repeating again and again, "Don't worry, honey! It's all good," or whatever particular slang you like to use. It may not feel like it at the moment, but this will become such second nature that you could do it with your eyes closed. Or at least with one eye on the TV. Which I've done (sorry, honey).

So, let's prep our patient, shall we? Most of the time the shot is given in the lower stomach, although sometimes it can be given in the leg or the arm (this is one of the few ex-ceptions to the "only in the stomach" rule). Personally, I say go for the stomach; it just seems to be the easiest place to do it. Depending on your wife's tolerance for pain, you may want to numb the area first. The best way I've found is a good old-fashioned ice cube. Yes, the old standby anesthetic for those junior high homemade ear piercings works just as well here.

While you prep the shot, give your wife an ice cube, and have her rub the area where the shot will go for five minutes or so. The skin will turn pink, which also gives you a good target area for your shot. And now, you're ready to . . .

STEP FOUR—Shoot it Up

This last step works best if your wife is lying down—on the bed, the couch, an ancient Japanese tatami mat. It doesn't matter. Your wife may or may not want to watch. If she watches it's not so much because she's utterly fascinated by the process, but more because she doesn't trust you. Personally, I say let her see it the first time—well, unless she's prone to throwing up or passing out—in which case just videotape it for future broadcast.

If your wife is anything like mine, one thing she'll definitely want to do is check your work. As in every single syringe, for the rest of the protocol. Again, it's only because she doesn't totally trust you. Chalk it up to that one time you arbitrarily decided to throw some cayenne and crushed red peppers into the pasta sauce you were making, just to "kick it up" a bit. They never seem to forget stuff like that, do they?

Still, we have to do what we have to do. So, now that we have the area icy and numb, let's do the do. Follow me, won't you?

1. Locate the pink, cold area on her stomach.

2. Take another alcohol pad and wipe the area. You can blow on it a couple of times to dry it off. Now you're ready.

3. Firmly grab the area in a pinch. I mean pinch *hard*. Yes, it will hurt her, but it will also distract her from the pain of the actual shot. It's an old trick invented by Chinese warlord Sun-Tzu. Or maybe it was David Copperfield. Either way, it works. Seriously, grab for whatever you can get: skin, fat, whatever. If she has a little bit of extra . . . well, *her* down there, all the better. Just don't mention it to her. *Ever*.

4. Holding the syringe like a dart, quickly bring the needle down into the pinched area, making sure not to move it *at all* once it's in. Seriously. It'll hurt. A lot.

5. Using your thumb, push down on the plunger slowly and evenly. Let it sit for a moment to make sure it's all out, and then pull the needle out on the *exact* same trajectory you used to put it in. There will probably be a drop of two of blood, so just dab it off.

6. Sit back and exhale. You're done.

Guess what? You just gave her a shot! You're *so* the man!

Oh, I almost forgot Step 7!: Cap the needle before you throw it away in the sharps container. You have no idea how many times you'll stab yourself when you forget to do that, especially once you start juggling three syringes a night. Surprisingly, the needles really hurt!

I should mention at this point that once it's inside of her, Lupron can be kind of . . . sting-y. She'll feel it start burning pretty fast, so be prepared to hear about it. There's really nothing you can do for her, so just deal. It's good prep for all of the complaints you'll be hearing about when she's pregnant, right?

Remember a little earlier when I compared giving your wife fertility injections to giving your wife "fertility injections"? (Yeah, that would be a sex reference, for the double-entendre impaired.) Well, it's actually true in a lot of ways. Take for example, the "overdoing it" factor. When it comes to sex, you need to change things up every once in a while. The same holds true with injections.

Each night you're going to have to alternate the sides where you give her the shot, and you'll also want to change the actual sites of the injections. A good rule of thumb is to work the area like a clock: start at one o'clock the first night, and then move clockwise each following night (still alternating sides, of course). By the time you get all the way around the "clock" to that first shot site, it should be *just* barely healed up enough for you to maul it again. As the ancient Greek Hippocrates—the father of modern medicine—once wrote, "Ain't the human body cool?"

Now even with your best efforts to alternate injection sites and sides, you're eventually going to run out of new places to inject her. Over the course of all of these shots, the whole area will become tender and possibly black-and-blue from all the abuse. She'll complain. You'll say, "Sorry, baby, nothing I can do," and then stick her again. She'll complain some more, and the majestic dance of life goes on. I just want you to know this is normal, you're not doing anything wrong, and there's really no way to prevent it from happening. All you can do is try using more ice and practicing your "sad, sympathetic face" in the mirror a few extra times a day. (NOTE: It really helps when you push your lower lip out a tad. If you can make it quiver just the *slightest* bit too, all the better.)

JAB!—JAB!—JAB!—BODY BLOW!— STIMULATE THOSE FOLLICLES

Just when you think you have the shot giving down to a science, it's time to introduce two new pointy little friends into the mix: your egg-follicle stimulating drugs. Yay. The thing about the follicle stimulating drugs is that your doctor never really knows exactly what's going to work. So, he usually suggests a cocktail. No, not *that* kind of cocktail. You know she can't have one of those—but *you* sure as hell can. In fact, you're probably in need of one right about now. I'm going to recommend a Cable Car, the signature drink at the Bellagio Hotel in Vegas, where Julie and I honeymooned:

½ oz Orange Curaçao liqueur

1 oz Captain Morgan Original Spiced Rum

½ oz lime juice

½ oz sweet-and-sour mix

Combine everything in a cocktail shaker with ice.
Shake well and strain into a chilled, sugar-rimmed
cocktail glass.

Seriously, it's *really* good. Just don't pound one before you give her the shots, huh?

No, for our purposes here, the cocktail consists of two or more types of FSH (follicle stimulating hormones), which combined with the Lupron, will hopefully make lots of little eggs for your doctor to choose from during the retrieval. (While these two new shots are obviously of the utmost importance, you'll also need to continue giving her small doses of Lupron in order to keep her ovulation suppressed during the rest of the cycle.)

The two most popular FSH concoctions are Menopur (pronounced MEN-oh-pure, just so you don't sound silly calling it Meno-purr or something like that) and Follistim (I'll assume you can pronounce that one). Your doctor may prescribe something else, but since this is what Julie and I used, plus I'm far too lazy to type up all the different drug names, we'll go with these.

FOLLISTIM

In a word, Follistim is frickin' awesome. Yeah, that's two words, but I'm giving it a bonus modifier for being so awesome. It's pretty much a completely self-contained system, and everything you need is all neatly packed together in one kit. Hey, they even give you this cool blue carrying case. And who doesn't like a blue carrying case, right?

If given the choice, always get the Follistim Pen. This is a really neat injection system that looks like, well, a pen (duh), but conceals the needle and drug safely inside. Seriously, this is real James Bond kind of stuff here: "See here, Bond—it looks like a pen, but when you take the cap off like so . . . you can get your wife pregnant."

The drugs themselves come in little cartridges that you put into the pen, and then you dial out a dosage. It's pretty much "Injections for Dummies," and man, I loved it! Actually, I let Julie do the dialing. That way she felt involved as well as secure in the knowledge that I wouldn't misjudge the dose and kill her. Did I mention your wife will constantly believe you're doing it wrong?

So, how do we use this incredible piece of space-age equipment? So glad you asked. Let's look at what you'll need:

- a Follistim pen

- a Follistim cartridge

- a Follistim needle tip

- an alcohol pad

I have to tell you that when you put this thing together you'll feel like one of those guys field stripping a rifle in a war movie. It's actually very cool and feels pretty satisfying when you finally "lock and load" the thing. Really, it does.

Okay, so here we go:

1. Take the Follistim cartridge from the packet. It kind of looks like one of those cologne testers you get at Macy's—if you get cologne testers at Macy's, I mean.

2. Using the alcohol pad, wipe the top of the cartridge. You only have to do this once per cartridge, because there are a few days' worth of drugs in there. This saves you many, many precious seconds, which you can use however you want. Why not take up an instrument?

3. Open up the pen by unscrewing the top, insert the cartridge just like you'd replace an ink cartridge in a refillable pen (make sure you have the correct side down), and then screw the top on again.

4. Use the alcohol wipe to clean off the little pad at the top of the pen. This one you'll have to do before

each shot, so you'll only have time to learn one instrument. Sorry.

5. Pull out one of the needle tips and *carefully* screw one into the tip of the pen, pushing the bottom of the needle through the pad.

6. Dial the pen to the correct injection amount (no, I'm not just babbling—your doctor will tell you what this means), and then prime the pen by pressing *just a little* on the plunger to get a drop at the tip of the needle.

Okay, so put that one off to the side for a minute, as now you'll get the final shot (whew!) ready.

MENOPUR

Not all of the gonadotropins you are given are premixed like the Follistim. Some are handed to you in a highly concentrated form—concentrated as in "pure uncut powder" that comes in its own vial and that you have to mix up yourself. Don't panic, though, it's easy . . . well, as long as you don't mess it up.

So here's what you need to mix up your little Menopur shot:

- the prepackaged syringe with the ½ inch needle

- the "big" needle—1 ½ inches and used *only* for mixing, *not* for actually giving the shot (once you see it, you'll know why—this thing could be loaded into an RPG and used as antitank ordinance)

- two vials—one of the Menopur powder, and one of saline water

- the ubiquitous alcohol pads

Ready to tackle the most complicated of the shots? Too bad, because we're doing it anyway, taking it step by step. And remember the two most important words right now are "don't panic" (closely followed by the next two most important words: "back rub"). Here we go:

1. Uncap both vials, and then, using the alcohol pad, sterilize both tops.

2. *Carefully* remove the small needle from the top of the syringe (keep the cap on), and *carefully* screw on the big needle. (IMPORTANT NOTE: Again, *do not* give the injection with this needle or your wife will kill you and never tell anyone where she buried the body.)

3. Push the needle into the *saline* vial and withdraw the correct amount of saline. (Your doctor will tell you how much. Pay attention.)

4. Withdraw that needle and then push it into the Menopur vial and squirt that sucker full of water. Now *swirl* the vial to mix the two. *Do not shake it.* You're trying to make a baby, not a martini.

5. Draw the correct amount of Menopur solution back into the syringe.

6. *Carefully* cap the big needle, take it off, and then replace the smaller needle again.

7. Hold it up to the light and depress the syringe slightly to get any air out. There should be a small droplet at the tip of the needle.

Guess what? You're done. Good news: You are now the proud owner of two syringes full of fertility medications. Bad news: It's time to get them from the syringe into your wife.

I'LL TAKE TWO SHOTS WITH A LUPRON CHASER, PLEASE

Okay, basically you're going to be giving these to her the same way you gave her the solo Lupron shots (see above). I can't stress the "ice cube step" enough. Number one rule here is the number, the better.

The order I used when giving Julie the three shots went like this: Follistim, Menopur, Lupron. Of the three, Menopur and Lupron will *sting* like a sum'bitch. Not too surprising, actually, when you think about the fact that Menopur is one of those lovely urinary-based gonadotropins (see chapter 5). Kinda makes sense that it would sting a wee bit. Yeah, sure, at first she'll complain a little, but give her some time; eventually, after a few weeks of this, she'll be complaining a *lot*.

You may wonder how, being the sensitive man and partner you are, you should be reacting to these constant moans of discomfort. Of course, as a good husband you just kiss her and tell her how proud you are of her to go through all of this, how brave she is, etc. From my own personal experience, it definitely helps you to be more convincing if you actually mean what you say to her. If it happens that you're just one of those guys who're not so good with words, then you can just stroke her hair and smile tenderly. But you should still try to work on your "tender smile." You'll need to be *really* good at it soon.

As you give her the shots, once again you should work in a circular pattern on her lower stomach, but still be aware that even if you do, she'll eventually be bruised beyond belief down there. Seriously, it'll look like she just did some ab work with Evander Holyfield. That's okay; it's normal. Besides, it's nothing compared to what her ass is going to look like once you start the progesterone!

PULL THAT TRIGGER

You made it! You finally reached the time of retrieval, and now there's one important shot you'll need to give her just once: the trigger shot. This is a syringe full of hCG (human chorionic gonadotropin), which, when injected, starts the hormonal rush causing her eggs to release within eighteen to thirty-six hours, at which point your doctor harvests them, and, hopefully, turns them into your future son or daughter. Now, at first glance, this will appear to be an even easier shot to give her than the Lupron: In fact, most of these trigger shots already come premixed *and* preloaded into the syringe. You literally just tear it open and pop it into her.

Ah, but here's the difference: You're now at that stage in the protocol where injections into the stomach just aren't going to cut it. Those shots were just a warm-up, the farm team, if you will. At this point, you've been called up to the majors, specifically, the *intramuscular* league. Yes, beginning with this injection (that's right—there's only one hCG shot, but that in no way means this will necessarily be the *last* shot), you're going to need to go *past* the skin and fat, and deep into *muscle tissue*—and quite frankly, the biggest mass of muscle tissue in the human body is . . . well, you're sitting on it.

Yes, you're about to become intimately involved with your wife's ass in a way neither you, nor she, ever could have imagined.

BUTT, I THOUGHT
I WAS SUPPOSED TO USE ICE?

Now when you were shoving a needle just into the top few layers of skin, ice worked just fine: It numbed the area nicely, so she couldn't feel a thing. Supposedly. When you're dealing with a hunk of muscle tissue like your butt, numbing is going to be out of the question.

Oh, sure, you could have her sit through all nine hours of *The Lord of the Rings* trilogy on DVD, but that would be a hassle every night. No, what you need to do is *relax* the muscle enough for the shot to hurt less. And what relaxes more than heat? Yes, a hot water bottle or a heating pad applied to her gluteus for a few minutes before the shots does a pretty good job of loosening up her buns enough for Mr. Needle's nightly visit.

The trigger shot is good practice, but after the transfer, she's going to be dropping trou on a nightly basis for the big daddy of all fertility injections (cue dramatic music): Progesterone!

PROGESTERONE

Now because both the flood of hormone injections into your wife's system plus the act of retrieving her eggs interfere with her natural progesterone production, your wife is going to need extra progesterone to make sure her uterus gets nice and sticky for the little sucker to implant. This usually lasts until about twelve weeks after the transfer of the embryos (the doctors like to be sure).

This extra progesterone, sometimes called PIO (*progesterone in oil*), is a thick, oily (obviously) liquid that you'll need to shoot into her butt every night. This is going to be a true test of your shot-giving skills, because everything is bigger and badder: The fluid is thicker, the needle is bigger, and her butt is sorer.

The easiest way to do this (as if there is one), is for you or the nurse at the clinic to take a heavy permanent marker and draw two largish circles about hip level on her butt cheeks, one on each side. Then, starting at the twelve o'clock position, inject her on alternate sides every night, making a daily rotation around her "moon."

Because the progesterone is suspended in a heavy oil, pushing down on that plunger is going to be a lot harder, which, in turn, makes it a lot harder to keep the needle steady. And you'd better keep it steady. Julie could feel if its trajectory was off by a micrometer once it hit her ass. A fair warning that when it comes to giving this shot, there's going to be a lot of yelling, screaming, and possibly even crying. Your wife might do some too.

Now, if you want to be a hero, or even just *look* like one, suggest to your wife that she think about trying *ethyl oleate*. This is a medium that is thinner than oil and that, in general, women find hurts a lot less. Picture pushing down on a syringe filled with caramel vs. one filled with lemonade. I think you can appreciate why she'd prefer the ethyl oleate. Now she'll probably already know about this, because every woman on the online message boards knows about this, but you'll look like a stud if you just *happen* to mention this out of the blue. Extra points if you do it in front of your doctor!

Another warning: If you love—I mean *really* love—looking at your wife's beautiful ass, then you'd best take a picture of it and turn it into your screensaver, because with one of these bad boys a day every day for twelve weeks you're going to see the kind of bruising that would put Rocky Balboa's mug to shame. On the other hand, if purple is her color, it might be a good look for her.

THE UPSIDE

Congratulations! You now know all there is to know about giving your wife fertility injections. What do you get out of this? Well, a few things, all of them good.

For one, you're playing a monumental role in the creation of your child. Sure, any guy can masturbate into a cup, but you—you acted like a man and gave her the shots she needed to sustain your child's life. Besides, could you imagine her twisting herself around to give herself those shots in the butt? Not a pretty picture.

Also, you're going to come off as a *massive* hero here. When she tells her friends about her experience (and you know she will), she's going to let all of them know how you bravely dealt with the needle issue. And then her friends, being impressed, will tell their husbands, who will look upon you as a pseudodeity and construct shrines and hold great feasts in your honor. Well, at least they'll think you're a pretty badass hombre.

TEN

Okay, Seriously,
This $#!%
Ain't Working!

*N*ow, because fertility treatments are an art just as much as a science, just like art, what works for some people doesn't always work for others. And, unfortunately, it's at this point that you may find yourself grouped into that "others" category. It may be the fault of the doctor, who fails to adjust the treatments each cycle—or it may not. It may be the fault of the parents, who just don't have "the right stuff" for conception—or it may not. It may come down to nothing more than bad chemistry, and things just don't gel together the way they're supposed to. In any case, you may very well find yourselves having to decide if you should continue down the road of IVF treatments, or move on to other methods.

HEY, NICE PACKAGE!

If your fertility doctor is like my fertility doctor (it could be the same guy for all I know; if it is, say hi for me, would you?), then he or she offers a package plan for fertility treatments. What does that mean? It means instead of one cycle for one price, you can buy two or three cycles and pay for them up front, at a reduced price of course. Is this a good idea? Well, it depends. You need to take into account the fact that very few fertility cycles work that first time, which means that you may be looking at a couple, or more than a couple, tries. Obviously that can turn into some big bucks. As in "luxury car" kind of money—minus the GPS and DVD setup. But as far as those two options go: 1) you're a guy; you don't need a map because you just drive around the general area till you eventually find where you're going, and 2) you shouldn't be watching TV in the car anyway.

Sure, you can balk at the cash, but before you start your balking, think about this: If it turns out the first cycle *doesn't* work, and you and your wife are faced with the emotional turmoil that will almost certainly follow afterward, wouldn't you rather take some small comfort knowing your next cycle is already bought and paid for, sitting there and waiting for when you two are ready for another shot? Or would you feel better realizing that if you wanted to take another grab at the brass ring, you'd have to pay full price? When you buy life insurance, the irony is that you pay for it year after year, all the while praying you'll never need it. With the IVF package deals, consider them to be a kind of "fertility insurance": Sure, if you're lucky you'll never need it, but it's a good thing to know it's there if you do.

Or, you may want to take a trip down to the bank ...

NOW THAT'S SOME SPERM
YOU CAN BANK ON!

Ah, the sperm bank. The punch line of a thousand dirty jokes. The jumping-off point of a hundred terrible TV movies. It does exist though, and it exists for a reason: Sometimes, our sperm just plain sucks.

You remember how we talked about sperm motility and morphology and all of those great ways to measure your swimmers, right? I'll assume you do. Now, if there are problems with either the movement or the shape of your sperm, modern science has techniques that can help you out.

One example is ICSI (pronounced ICK-see), which stands for *intracytoplasmic sperm injection*. It's a state-of-the-art micromanipulation technique (which means that lab techs can do things under a microscope using tiny precision tools that would be impossible for an unaided human to accomplish; in other words, it's not easy at all). In ICSI, individual sperm cells are injected *right into the egg*, which is really amazing, especially if you're not into all that messy *sex* stuff.

On the other hand, some men have no live sperm at all. Seriously. In cases like that, it's necessary to find some "third-party sperm." It can come from a variety of sources, but usually it is either donated by someone you know (which definitely opens the door to about seventeen different kinds of creepy), or you pick the donor from a sperm bank.

The good thing about the sperm bank option is that you get to choose the sperm you want to use. Well, technically, you get to choose the sperm *donor*; it would take far too long to do it the other way. Oh, and contrary to what those crap comedy movies would have you believe, there are actually qualifications donors need to have in order to donate:

- Height: between 5'10" and 6' tall (people want small babies, not small children).

- Weight: proportionate to height (so no pro wrestlers need apply—sorry guys).

- Education: college educated at least, advanced degrees are preferred (yes, it takes a genius to masturbate into a cup these days).

- Age: prime fertility age of nineteen to thirty-nine (nobody wants old, decrepit sperm—sorry 'bout that, Hef—you still put out a fine magazine, though).

- Sperm screening: for any diseases, genetic abnormalities, etc. (no bad seed is getting through these filters!).

Needless to say, the sperm you're getting from a bank is top-notch, with high motility and morphology. If you're spending money on the product, the bank wants you to know that it's got a good shot at working.

Once you've picked out your donor, the rest is cake: The spermcicle is taken from the bank, thawed, and then inserted into the uterus just as if it were a normal IUI. If the problem was simply a male-factor issue, this has a very good chance of working. But what if we're putting the sperm before the egg, so to speak?

"WHILE YOU'RE OUT, CAN YOU GRAB US SOME EGGS?"

Sperm isn't the only thing that can be donated by outside sources. In some cases, it's the woman's eggs that are, to put it in the parlance of those old, embarrassing commercials, "not so fresh" (i.e., her eggs are no good).

Up until recently, if a woman had poor-quality eggs, or worse yet, if she had no eggs at all, pretty much the only option was to look up the number of a good adoption agency. Not so much now. What changed? Three little letters: IVF. Remember, in vitro fertilization involves the implantation of a fertilized egg in a woman's uterus. Notice I said "a fertilized egg," not "her fertilized egg." Bling! Lights just went on, didn't they?

In the case of using a donor egg, it's the husband's sperm being used to fertilize a "third-party egg." Now you may be questioning how an egg would get donated in the first place. Good question. It means you're paying attention. Okay, let's look at a few ways the egg could get from "Woman A" to "Point B":

- You can use a friend or relative. (By relative I assume you know I mean "her" relative, not yours, unless you're looking to play Deliverance: The Home Game.)

- There are women who are either paid to donate eggs or who do so voluntarily at your fertility clinic.

(These women are, both literally and figuratively, "good eggs." Sorry.)

- There are private brokers you can use who specialize in setting up donors with needy couples. (In these cases, it's very, very important to get legal help in drawing up the contracts. When it comes to future children, you want to leave *nothing* to chance.)

In the first case above (the friend or relative), the donor has to realize she's taking on a huge responsibility. It's not just a matter of knocking on your friend's door and asking to borrow a couple of eggs. Oh, no. They have to go through the whole cycle of injections needed to prep the eggs for retrieval just like someone getting ready for IVF (see chapter 9).

Another problem comes in the realization that, just like in a regular IVF cycle, you will have no idea how many eggs your volunteer will actually come up with. If she doesn't respond well to the hormones, it could be very few, if any at all. No guarantees at all on this one.

In addition, cost is going to be a factor. Yes, just like at the market, grade-A eggs are sold at a premium. Why? Well, think about it: A man has millions and millions of sperm, and to get them out, well, it's not the hardest thing in the world. Hell, we can do it in our sleep (and plenty of us do!). Eggs? Well, they're another story.

Eggs take a lot to prep and extract, and women who do this expect to be compensated. Women with really good genes and high IQs who made All State in women's volleyball during college and went on to become lawyers don't just grow on trees, so they expect to be compensated a *lot*. How much? Let's just say a whole lot more than a "normal" donor, as in thousands of dollars *per egg*. But really, how much would you be willing to pay for a kid with a really great downward spike?

I'D LIKE TO RENT A WOMB
FOR NINE MONTHS, PLEASE . . .

Okay, so suppose you have an egg and a sperm that are good, but your wife's uterus isn't capable of maintaining the pregnancy. In that case, you simply go out and rent a surrogate womb.

That sounded cruder than it actually is. What you're doing is going through the whole IVF cycle as outlined in chapter 6, but when it comes time to implant the embryo, you're just implanting it in a third party. A really generous third party, who doesn't mind going through the whole pregnancy for a child who isn't genetically hers in the least.

This is another circumstance when you might want to ask a friend or relative to, as the Beatles so lyrically put it, "Carry that weight for a long time." Since there's no true DNA comingling, you're not going to get any of those pesky genetic abnormalities, plus you would have full access to the person in order to monitor the pregnancy as much as you like.

In the event that you can't find a friend or relative, yes, there are women who do this for a living, or at least do it to make extra money. As hard as I found this to believe when I first heard it, some women *love* being pregnant. Like really, *really* love it. For them, going through the joy of pregnancy without having to take care of the baby afterward is like eating a hot fudge sundae without getting the calories, except that there's more bleeding involved. With the birth, I mean, not the sundaes.

The downside? There're a few. For one, no matter whom the baby belongs to genetically, the law states that the surrogate carrier ultimately has control over any testing or decisions to abort the pregnancy, so you better have an ironclad legal agreement if you want to circumvent these problems. Also, there are a lot of scummy people out there who live to take advantage of couples grasping at their last chance to have a child. Sure, one day those people are going to have their own intestines fed to them while they burn in the deepest, darkest pits of hell, but in the meantime, be very careful in selecting a donor womb, and for God's sake get yourself a lawyer (he'll probably be burning in the deepest, darkest pits of hell too, but for something entirely different).

SURROGATE CITY

Now if your wife's eggs *and* womb are both problematic—a very gentle euphemism in the world of infertility, lemme tell you!—there's also the option of what's commonly thought of as a "usual surrogate," in which a woman (not your wife) has your sperm implanted inside of her. It's done through an IUI and she then carries the baby to term. It's basically the opposite of the sperm donor situation, as the child will be genetically half yours (your sperm) and half the surrogate's (her egg), so all the same caveats apply: Screen the donor, make sure everything's legal, tax and license extra, your mileage may vary, etc.

HOW MUCH IS THAT
EMBRYO IN THE WINDOW?

The final genetic option available is a real doozy—donor embryos. Yep, medical science has taken the hard part out of actually creating an embryo for you, and now all you need to do is carry it to term! Easy! Well, not really . . .

Sometimes it happens that for whatever reason, even traditional IVF doesn't work on the genetic level. No matter how many eggs are injected with how many sperm in how many labs by how many doctors, that spark of life never ignites, and no embryos are ever formed. This is where the miracle of donor embryos comes in. It's an adoption done at the microgenetic level, so while your wife may be the one giving birth, genetically it will still be another couple's child.

Many couples who have had successful IVF cycles find they have to limit the number of embryos they can implant, even if they produced a good number that matured in the lab. So, what does one do with the extra embryos? Many couples opt to donate them to the clinic specifically for use as donor embryos for couples who aren't as lucky.

So, let's do the upside and downside again. The upside? You get to find out who the mother and father were, so it helps you "pick out" your embryo. That way, if you ever wanted a kid who was the genetic offspring of a Nobel Prize–winning doctor and a high-fashion supermodel, you could implant that specific embryo—well, assuming a Nobel Prize–winning doctor and a high-fashion supermodel got together, did IVF, and then donated their embryos to your clinic. It could happen . . .

Also, it's a compromise for couples who feel too awkward about using either donor sperm or eggs, since with donor embryos, it isn't one parent or the other who is genetically "left out." It's both of them.

The downside? It's a new science, and as such, the long-term effects haven't been studied. Also, legally it's uncharted territory. No one knows if in the future, genetic parents will be granted any rights to their "adopted" children. But, if you're willing to take the risk, I say go for it. I'm very supportive like that.

As you can see, no matter what your fertility issue might be, science (and caring donors and surrogates) can offer you hope. While you may not be creating your child in what is traditionally referred to as the "natural" way, you *are* creating *your* child, and in the end, that is all that matters.

ELEVEN

RE: Your Choice of
Fertility Doctor

*O*kay, so now you know a lot of what goes into fertility treatments. But before you start any of them up, you need to find a doctor, right? Well, unless you have a cousin who's looking to unload a whole crate of Menopur in a hurry ("What? It fell off a truck!"), then yeah, you need to find a fertility doctor, technically known as a *reproductive endocrinologist* (or RE for short). But where do you find them? What do you do once you find them? What if you don't like the one you find? If your mind is spinning with these questions, then spin no more.

IF YOU'RE FEELING INFERTILE/DON'T CRY OR SAY MAYBE/CALL DR. GOLDSTEIN/ HE'LL GIVE YOU THAT BABY! (*SE HABLA ESPAÑOL!*)

Let's say you're in the market for a new car. What do you do? Do you go out and buy the first car you see with a FOR SALE sign on the windshield? Of course not! Do you pick up the classified section of the newspaper, call up a number, and give the guy who picks up the phone your credit card number to buy his POS car sight unseen? Nope! Oh, maybe you go down to the car lot and pick out a new car and pay the first price the salesman quotes you. Are you insane?

When you and your wife find yourselves in the market for an RE, keep in mind that you're shopping for something that is quite a bit more important than a new car—and possibly much more expensive! But how do you pick out a fertility doctor? It's going to be a different method than just finding a general practitioner in the yellow pages. I mean they don't just take your temperature and read your blood pressure. Your fertility doctor has to help you make a baby! No, for something that important, you're going to need to know a bit more about him or her than whether or not they can come up with a catchy tagline for their phonebook ad.

So let's take a look at how you can find yourself the doctor of your dreams.

IF YOU DON'T ASK, NO ONE CAN TELL

I know it sounds very basic, but you should ask around. A few years ago, infertility was something that was spoken of in hushed voices, a shame that earned you and your wife a scarlet letter. Maybe even two—you know, so you guys can match. These days, with celebrities doing it, reality shows with multiple births from fertility medications, etc., it's as common as an everyday run-of-the-mill nose job—well, maybe a really long, *involved* nose job that lasts several months . . . and ends with a baby coming out of her nostril . . . Alright, maybe not the best analogy, but you see what I'm getting at: Infertility and its treatments are a lot more common and a lot less shocking nowadays.

That being said, if you feel comfortable enough, you should literally ask around. I'm guaranteeing you right now that someone you know knows someone who has either gone through what you're going through, or is going through it right now. Julie and I were shocked at how many times we met people who, once we mentioned our fertility treatments, suddenly let loose a river of stories about their cousin Yitzik (probably not his real name) whose wife is going through their third IVF treatment, and how *great* their doctor is, and how you should definitely give him a call, etc.

Word-of-mouth is a major way many fertility practices grow their businesses. After all, if you can get a good recommendation about one doctor versus another, chances are you'd go with it, right?

REFER MADNESS

Looking for something a bit more reliable than word-of-mouth or hearsay? How about a good old-fashioned doctor's referral? Julie and I went this route. Early on in our frustration, Julie went in to see her gynecologist—before we figured out that I was the one with the problem. After giving her the once-over, he suggested we go talk to a fertility doctor. In fact, being something of a big shot at Cedars-Sinai Hospital, he was able to give us a referral to one of the top REs in Los Angeles. Yippee!

Of course, you don't need to come to Los Angeles to see a good RE. Fertility clinics can be found in almost every one of the United States, as well as in countries as far away and exotic as Australia, Egypt, and Barbados. Your wife has a good relationship with her gynecologist (at least I hope so, considering what he or she is doing down there!), so they are an excellent place to start collecting names and references.

When you do get a referral, try to suss out from your doctor *why* he or she referred you to that particular RE. Is it because they have a great record and come highly recommended by former patients or is it because they have some kind of shady payoff tit-for-tat referral deal? Not that I'm trying to impugn your wife's doctor. He may be a perfectly lovely person who gives to charity and cherishes birds and spiders and all other living things—but it never hurts to ask, right?

NUMBER CRUNCHING BY THE NUMBERS

You have the name of a doctor. Hopefully you have a few. Fantastic. Now, whom do you use? While I'm sure you have several tried-and-true methods for picking something you know nothing about—choosing a name blindly from a hat, eeny meeny miny moe, darts—might I suggest a more reliable alternative?

We live in a wondrous time when every bit of information you can possibly ask for is literally at your fingertips on the Internet. There's even a site you can use to compare fertility doctors: www.CDC.gov. Now, as you can see from the address, it *is* run by the U.S. government, specifically the Centers for Disease Control, but don't let that stop you, since the methods they use are verifiable and reliable.

Each year, the CDC compiles a list of fertility clinic data, sort of a Consumer Reports survey, only instead of washing machines and cell phones, it looks at REs and their statistics: How many fertility treatments does the clinic perform each year? How many cycles are canceled because they did not work? And most importantly, what is the clinic's live birth rate? The live birth rate is defined as the number of fertility cycles that lead to an *actual live birth* of a baby.

This is the big number you need to look at, because obviously this is what it's all about. If a clinic does hundreds of cycles but has a very low live birth rate percentage number, then that's obviously not the one you want to go to. Factory-style assembly lines are good for making subcompact cars, not babies.

Also, like the old hackneyed real estate joke goes, one of the most important things about your fertility clinic is *location, location, location*. Realize that when you're in the middle of a fertility treatment, you or your wife (perhaps both of you) are going to have to go to the clinic a few times a week. If the one you think you like turns out to be a two-and-a-half-hour plane ride away, well, perhaps that's a commute you're not ready to commit to—unless you really like those tiny airline bags of honey-roasted peanuts, in which case, the choice is entirely up to you. I'm only here to help.

Once you've narrowed it down to one or two likely candidates, it's time to meet your prospective doctors . . .

YOU CAN'T ALWAYS JUDGE A CLINIC
BY ITS MAGAZINES

The first time Julie and I went to see our RE I have to admit I was impressed. Located in the heart of Beverly Hills, this was the fertility clinic to end all fertility clinics. We've all seen the TV shows set in a ritzy doctor's office, with the chic glass walls and fine calfskin couches and designer coffee tables brimming with magazines published within the last month, flat panel LCD TVs mounted all over the waiting room, and the ferns . . . my God, the ferns! Add to that a huge wall covered with pictures and holiday cards showing happy families, all from parents professing gushing, heartfelt thanks to the doctor for making their dreams come true and giving them the children they so desperately wanted but could never have. Damn. I was in.

Being a guy, I was most impressed with the amount and expense of their toys. Julie, on the other hand, had actual questions for the doctor. Unless you've done a lot of research beforehand (and, what with you being the husband, most likely you haven't) you'll want to follow your wife's lead on this one. She's been on the Web sites. She's talked to the former patients. She's already pre-filled out the forms. She's the woman in the know.

That does *not* mean, however, that once you walk into the doctor's office you just sit down, nod your head, and grin like Chucko the Idiot Monkey Boy. You're an integral part of this operation, and you've got questions too . . . You just don't know what they are yet.

If, when you sit down with the doctor, he opens the meeting by saying, "So, what brings you here?" Get up and run away. Hopefully, the doctor has done some kind of prep work and read your file, seen your concerns, and has at least some idea of possible treatments for you. Of course, he won't know any of the details until he gets your tests back, but a good RE can look at symptoms and get a ballpark idea of what he's dealing with. With experience comes wisdom. It's like how a good dry cleaner can look at a stain and know what he's going to need to get it out without having all the details as to how that much blood got on your suit jacket in the first place.

LET'S PLAY TWENTY QUESTIONS.
MAYBE THIRTY QUESTIONS.
OKAY, FORTY QUESTIONS.

After your doctor has looked at your test results, he or she will have a much better idea of what kinds of protocols would have the greatest chance of working for you. Now is the time for the in-depth questions. Of course, hopefully after reading this book you won't have too many, but maybe that's just wishful thinking on my part. After all, if you're making this kind of investment in blood, sweat, and tears—not to mention cash—you have every right to ask as many questions as you want to.

That's actually a good first test of the doctor. If he's not into answering your questions, or just blows you off, he's probably not the right guy for you. Yes, it's all fine and good that he knows what he's doing (you hope!), but it's equally important that *you* know what he's doing, and why.

SO . . . CAN I CALL YOU LATER?

Another very important thing to consider when picking a doctor is communication. As I said, it's a really good idea if the doctor can explain what he's doing and why in a way that you'll understand. Another good quality for your potential RE to have is an openness to communicate with you.

When Julie and I started our first IVF protocol, we quickly found out we had questions even after we met with the doctor. After all, I was sticking needles in her and injecting her with massive amounts of hormones. She started feeling weird, then weird turned into sick, which then morphed into what I could only charitably describe as "psychopathic rage." Naturally I was concerned.

We tried calling our doctor at the clinic, but found him less than responsive. Basically, after the first couple of times we met with him, he suddenly became like the voice in the box from *Charlie's Angels*. He was mysterious, rarely called us back, and in all likelihood was off cavorting in Saint-Tropez with some hot blonde. Okay, maybe not so much that last one, but he was a hard man to nail down.

Sure, we talked to nurses and support staff, but we really wanted to speak to the *doctor* directly. We realized he had a lot of other patients—hey, those ferns didn't pay for themselves—but as far as we were concerned, we should be his number one priority! And even if we weren't, couldn't he at least pretend we were? We were easy. We could accept a lie.

What's worse, when we finished our first cycle, and it turned out to be negative, we did finally get a phone call from him, but he sounded so detached and clinical that he might as well have been someone calling from the power company telling us our electric bill was overdue. I mean really, all of our hopes and dreams we had been focused on for weeks and weeks had just been crushed into oblivion, and all he did was shrug (granted, it was over the phone, but it *sounded* like a shrug—I'm pretty sure I heard his jacket crinkle) and say, "Well, we can always try it again." Look, we knew this was his job, and he probably has to make lots of bad, and good, calls every day, but the fact that he didn't really take our feelings into account was a definite black mark in our book.

What we found out the hard way, and what you're going to want to find out from the doctor ahead of time, is exactly what lines of communication he or she plans to keep open. Are they so busy that they will simply relegate any questions to their support staff, or are they really involved and don't mind a bit of hand-holding as newbies go through the process? Depending on how confident or nervous you are about the protocol, that can make a huge difference.

ABANDON SHIP!

Depending on how well your treatment works, there may come a time—as was the case with us—where you feel that this one particular doctor is just not meeting your needs. The question then arises: Do we stop, or do we find another doctor?

It was after our third IVF cycle, and our fourth try overall. After our doctor's fourth shrugging of the shoulders (by this time I was *sure* he was doing that!), Julie and I looked at one another and said, "This is ridiculous." Here we were killing ourselves with all of these shots and hormones, over and over again, only to feel the heartbreak of finding out it was all for nothing. What were we doing to ourselves? This was no way to live our lives.

We really, truly were ready to give up and look into some alternative way of having a child, maybe adopting, when purely by chance Julie went to a party and met a friend of a friend who had just gone through a successful cycle with another fertility doctor. Now this friend couldn't stop raving about this RE, so Julie and I looked at each other again (we do like looking at each other a lot, don't we?) and said, "One more try."

We went to this doctor's office, and really, it couldn't have been more different. Instead of chic and tony Beverly Hills, we found ourselves deep in the San Fernando Valley. No flat panel TVs on the office walls, no calfskin sofas, and certainly no ferns. (Though to be fair, the magazines were still pretty much current, so I wasn't completely scared off.)

We sat down with the doctor, and immediately we knew we liked this guy. He was boisterous and funny—and confident. Damn was he confident, bordering on cocky. He flipped through our file, looking at what our previous doctor did, and then looked up at us and almost casually said, "Oh, yeah, I know what we need to do. I'm sure this time we'll get you your baby." Holy shit! Are you kidding me? But I was sold.

We went through the IVF protocol, and the amazing thing was that when we had questions—and yes, even the fifth time around, you will have questions—he was actually available! When we needed to speak to the doctor, we spoke to the doctor. This blew our minds.

But what was *really* amazing was when we found out our doctor's confidence wasn't just egotistical bullshit. Sure enough, he did get us our baby. *On the first try.* Well, the first try with him, anyway. Now it was our turn to gush to him about how he made all our dreams come true by giving us the child we thought we could never have. And all because we decided to try that one more time.

The moral of the story is that just because one doctor doesn't work, it doesn't mean there aren't any fertility treatments that will. Sometimes, as in our case, it takes a pair of fresh eyes, or a different attitude, or a smaller practice—whatever. I keep repeating that fertility treatments are an art, but that's because they really, truly are. If one artist doesn't have the vision to see David standing there in that big block of marble, then you go and find yourself another sculptor who can.

(NOTE: Just as an aside, in the course of researching this book, I happened to stop back in to our second RE's office a few months ago, and *wow!* Talk about redecorating! I'm talking big ol' plasma screens set into the walls, a sweet new glass conference room ... so okay, maybe the *secondary* moral to this story is that while you shouldn't judge a book by its cover, a nice, shiny dust jacket can definitely make you want to flip through the pages.)

Okay, so now you have a doctor, and you have a prescribed protocol. But IVF medication doesn't grow on trees, and most clinics aren't running on smiles, rainbows, and gumdrops. And even if they were, gumdrops still cost money. What I'm getting at is exactly how are you planning to pay for this endeavor?

In the next chapter, we'll take a look at some of your options, and you do have a few.

TWELVE

So Will You Be Using Cash, Credit, or Your Home Equity Line?

*C*ontrary to popular myth, babies aren't delivered by storks. I'll assume you know that, and if you don't, might I suggest you check out some more remedial books before finishing this one? The technology of ART (IUIs, IVFs, etc.) is highly specialized, and working with genetics on the level that the REs do requires a great deal of equipment and skill. It can cost millions of dollars just to set up the lab where your future child will be cultivated. That's a hell of a start-up cost.

In a nutshell, ART is expensive. We're talking anywhere from a few grand to tens of thousands of dollars. Yeah. So after you've done all the research, read all the books, visited all the clinics, and met with all of the doctors, the inevitable question arises: "How the hell are we going to pay for all of this?"

INSURANCE: THE BEST POLICY YOU CAN HAVE NEXT TO HONESTY

Usually, when we're talking about expensive medical procedures, the first thing you think about is our old friend health insurance. The good news about insurance is that nearly everyone in the United States is covered by some kind of policy, either privately, corporately, or through the government.

The bad news is that benefits offered by insurance companies in regard to fertility treatments can vary as wildly as the Dodgers' playing skills whenever they make it into the playoffs. In fact, many of the insurance companies that do offer benefits only do so because they are required to by individual states, and even then chances are those benefits aren't to the extent that you'll need them.

WHAT'S THE STATE OF YOUR INSURANCE?

As of the writing of this book, there are fifteen states that mandate by law that insurance companies practicing within their borders must at least offer some form of fertility treatment coverage. Sounds good, right? Eh, not so fast. I don't know if anyone ever told you this, but those politicians—they tend to be a little tricky from time to time.

First of all, if you work for a company with over five hundred employees, the company's insurance carrier is exempt from having to follow these laws. Why? Because then the company is under federal regulation, instead of state regulation, and as of now there are no federal laws that require the coverage of fertility treatments. Unfortunately, that's one of the pitfalls of the American federalist system we all know and love.

Now, you'll notice I said the states mandate that insurance companies at least *offer* fertility coverage. In three of those fifteen states (California, Connecticut, and Texas), that means that all the insurance companies have to do is say to the employers buying insurance for their employees, "Hey, you want to buy fertility insurance for your people?" To which the employer is free to respond, "Nope. Now, about this 'alien attack' clause here . . ."

For the remaining twelve states (Arkansas, Hawaii, Illinois, Louisiana, Maryland, Massachusetts, Montana, Ohio, New Jersey, New York, Rhode Island, and West Virginia), state law says that while insurance companies must provide some form of fertility treatment insurance, it's up to each individual state to decide *how much* must be provided. Some can give you the full Monty (total, multiple IVF treatments), while some may just cover tests and medications. Go online and look into it or call your insurance company and check it out. But don't look a gift horse in the mouth; even if it's just a round of injectable medications that is covered, that's still a few thousand dollars in your pocket, and lemme tell you, strollers ain't cheap.

Oh, and one more *caveat* regarding going through insurance companies: Even if you do find yourself lucky enough to have some kind of fertility treatment coverage, you may have to choose your RE from your insurance company's "approved list" of doctors. And let me tell you, just because they've approved these doctors doesn't necessarily mean you will. They may be the ones who work the cheapest as far as the insurance reimbursement is concerned, but they may not be the best. And like I said in the previous chapter, choosing an RE that meshes well with you and your needs is of paramount importance.

GIVE ME SOME CREDIT!

If insurance is in no way, shape, or form an option, fear not. Well, I mean you can fear a little, but realize that there are, indeed, other options that might be available to you if you're intent on going through with fertility treatments.

Of course, the number one thing people think of is their credit card. Many people have credit limits far and above the amounts it would take to fund a fertility treatment, so it would seem an attractive choice for financing. Now, setting aside the well-known fact that credit card companies are actually subsidiaries of The Devil, Inc., and are, in fact, headquartered in the Ninth Circle of Hell, there are a few pros and cons to consider when paying with plastic.

- **Pro:** You can easily pay for your treatments in one lump amount, which, in some clinics, means a reduced rate.

- **Con:** You will then accrue interest on said lump amount at whatever rate your card charges. Now if you have a card that gives you a year at 0 percent, and you think you can pay this puppy off in twelve months or less, then awesome. If you have one of those cards where out of the blue they'll jack up your interest rate to 28 percent just because you looked at them funny, or if you think it's going to take you some time to pay off the balance, then you need to do some serious math. If you pay $10,000 at even 18

191

percent interest over three years, it means you're in for an extra $1,800. But sometimes you have to do what you have to do.

- **Pro:** If you get free stuff by using your card for "points" or "miles" or "credits" or whatever cute name the card company uses for its reward system, then you'll definitely be earning yourself a lot of said cutely named rewards.

- **Con:** If you do use your card, and you get a little . . . shall we say "lax," with the payments, then say bye-bye to your credit score, and to that quaint little future dream house with the lawn and the picket fence and the nosy but wacky neighbors where the two of you and your new bundle of joy will one day live happily ever after. Not trying to be a Debbie Downer, but someone has to say it: Sometimes when you want something as badly as you want this, you can lose sight of the facts, and credit problems are a fact.

So, does that mean you shouldn't ever use credit to pay for fertility treatments? Hell no! Truthfully, Julie and I ended up using a *whole lot* of it. One of our favorite games to play at the end of each month is Juggle the Cards, where we sit around the kitchen table to see which card we can pay off using a lower interest rate on another card. Fun for the whole family!

But let's just say that you don't want to go the credit route. Okay, well of course there are yet other options for you.

HOME SWEET HOME EQUITY

So, say you already have that dream house. Great! Say you're one of the lucky ones who have actually built up equity in your home. Awesome! Now you have yourself another option for getting money to fund your fertility treatments: the home equity loan.

Again, you have your pros and cons:

- **Pro:** You can take out a sizable chunk of change, which is good because you'll need it.

- **Con:** If you miss a payment, you could lose your home.

- **Pro:** The interest rate is pretty low, plus, since it's considered a second mortgage, you can deduct it at the end of the year.

- **Con:** If you miss a payment, *you could lose your home.*

At first glance, there seem to be more pros than cons, but that con is a big one. With the instability of the housing market, a lot of people who take out that second loan on their house quickly find themselves upside down and owing a lot more than their home is worth, and again, there go your dreams of returning at the end of a hard day to the wife and kids waiting for you *at home*.

EH, THOSE "GOLDEN YEARS" ARE OVERRATED ANYWAY

Now, there's always the possibility of cracking open your savings and/or retirement accounts, assuming you have either one. (Just as an aside, if you don't have at least a retirement account set up, you really should. Despite what it feels like right now, you won't be working forever, and those Del Webb communities aren't cheap.)

Of course if you have savings, you can dip into it—that's what it's there for, right? Sure, if you spend the vacation fund now you won't be taking that fabulous trip to Malaysia next year, but consider it this way: If everything goes well, in a few years you'll be taking the whole clan to Disney World, (What? Both places have pirates.)

Retirement accounts are a little trickier. IRAs and 401Ks can be dipped into or borrowed against, but remember, there are possible financial penalties involved. At first glance, these may sound like a deal, since your credit card interest rate is considerably higher than the normal 10 percent penalty for withdrawing funds from a 401K, but think a bit more. Remember, the 401K is made up of money that hasn't been taxed yet—but all that changes when you pull it out.

If you take money from the 401K, you are charged a 10 percent penalty fee *plus* the normal federal and state income taxes on the money. Ouch. "Okay," you say. "I'll just borrow against the 401K. That way I won't get dinged for the withdrawal." True. But you do need to repay the loan, and that extra money is going to be coming out of your paycheck, the same way your normal 401K contributions do. That means less take-home pay, which could (and will) be a hardship once the baby comes *and* you're still paying back the loan.

I'm not trying to dissuade you here—far from it. I just want you to go into this financing decision with both eyes open.

IF YOU ASK ME, THAT WHOLE "NEITHER A BORROWER NOR A LENDER BE" THING IS A LOAD OF CRAP

There is a type of loan that has the potential to be considerably less restrictive, yet infinitely more dangerous, than one from a bank: I am talking, of course, about the loan from your family and/or friends.

I will remind you at this point that what you're trying to get money for here isn't just some spur-of-the-moment itch or frivolous purchase. You and your wife are attempting to have a child, which will not only complete your family unit, but also give you a lifetime of joy. What does this mean? It means you shouldn't let something as petty as pride get in your way at this point.

A lot of people have a big problem with asking their friends and/or family for help. Our society says that if a man can't provide enough for his wife's needs, he's not a real man. You know what? "To provide" doesn't necessarily just mean to go out and hunt down a mastodon or to pull in the big bucks; it also means you will do everything in your power, moving heaven and earth, to get what she—and you—need. Sometimes that's as simple as asking someone for something.

Julie and I were extraordinarily lucky, since my family was in a position to help us out—repeatedly. While they are by no means wealthy, my mom and dad had some money put away, and they offered it to us. They explained that it was their joy to do this, since they wanted to have a grandchild to play with and spoil, and that it would give them more happiness than whatever possible retirement vacation they could buy with the same amount of money—and for that selflessness, we will be forever grateful.

Bruised egos aside, the old saw that "it never hurts to ask" holds true. Sure, your family may not be able to pitch in a huge amount, but a little something is better than nothing. Hell, be creative: Promise to name your firstborn after whoever gives the most. Though that may not be the best idea if you happen to have a wealthy great-uncle Blort.

LET'S MAKE A DEAL!

Aside from raising finances, you can sometimes get yourself a good deal from the clinic itself. As I mentioned in chapter 11, your clinic may offer you the equivalent of "buy one for $2, or three for $5" in that they'll give you a considerable discount on your fertility procedures if you buy two, three, or more cycles in advance. It's a rare hybrid of an investment/ gamble: If you go through your IVF cycle and it doesn't work, then hey, you've already got another paid-for cycle in the on-deck circle, ready for your next try. If it does work, then yes, you lose the money you've paid for the other cycles. But on the other hand you've got a baby to show for it, so in my mind it kind of evens out. And if that's not enough, some clinics even give you a partial refund if *none* of the cycles work, though that's small comfort considering what you were trying for. Check with your clinic for the exact details of what they offer.

There are other deals you can make as well, depending on your clinic. If you agree to be an embryo donor and allow your unused embryos to be frozen and used by couples who choose to go that route, sometimes clinics will give you a few thousand dollars off the price of your cycle. The downside is that if it works for them, one of your genetic offspring will be born and raised in a family of strangers. Some people can handle that thought, while others . . .

A FRAGMENT OF FINAL FINANCIAL PHILOSOPHY (TRY SAYING *THAT* FIVE TIMES FAST)

It's been said that the most common cause for stress in a marriage is money problems—followed closely by the "great toilet seat conundrum." Now, add these money problems to the stress of not being able to conceive normally, and you have enough to test even the strongest marriage. And I mean *test*. If you don't feel like you want to kill one another at least once during all of these fertility treatments, then please go to the Middle East and negotiate some treaties, because truly, your patience knows no bounds.

What the two of you need to do is sit down and have an honest, open discussion about your worries—both about the fertility treatments and the financial aspects thereof. I'll guarantee that both of you find out that the other one was holding back a lot of thoughts and fears that came out instead as hostility. You'll both feel a lot better, I promise you, and maybe you can even brainstorm a few new ideas on how to pay for this thing.

And above all, even though it sounds corny and you've heard it a million times, I want you to remember that if you really, truly want something badly enough, you'll find a way to make it happen. Unless what you want is a fast-food burger that looks like the one in the commercial. That just doesn't exist in our world, or any other. Sorry.

THIRTEEN

Finally!!

*E*veryone has a different way of finding out if it worked. Some actually wait for the doctor's office visit to take their official "Are we pregnant?" blood test. Most don't.

HEY, WHAT'D YOU GET ON THE TEST?

The night before our scheduled test with our fertility doctor, we were on pins and needles. We knew we had an appointment at nine o'clock the next morning, and we would get the results back from the blood test early that same afternoon. But we were so nervous! Would it work this time? What if it didn't? What if it's negative? What if whatever's wrong with us is impossible to fix? What if we just weren't supposed to have children?

Now, as I've mentioned, the one thing your doctor will tell you *not* to do is take a home pregnancy test before you take the official pregnancy blood test. The hormones that the blood test detects might still be too low to register on a store-bought test, and if you do end up with a false negative, you can plunge yourself into a monstrous, unwarranted depression. On the other hand, if you get a false positive, well, that could be even more horrible when you find out the truth.

And so, with this wise piece of advice from our doctor echoing in our ears . . . we raced out at ten o'clock that night to the nearest drugstore and bought a home pregnancy test.

Once we got home, we tore open the box like it was a Christmas present (technically, for us Hanukkah, but the analogy still applies). Even when the test stick was clear of the box, we still wondered: Should we really do this? Are we ready for whatever the result might turn out to be? Especially if it's a BFN—that's a "big fat negative" in fertility message board speak. And the worst part was, Julie was too nervous to pee. That's kind of important for a test that requires urine.

Finally, we swallowed our fear (and Julie swallowed a few cups of water), and she bravely strode into the bathroom, while I sat down on the couch and bravely turned on the TV. She finished and set it on the bathroom sink to set, or dry, or bake, or however these things work, and then came out. And we waited. We waited the longest three minutes of our lives. (Okay, technically we only waited two. If you haven't noticed by now, we're not exactly the most patient people when it comes to this stuff.) Finally, Julie took a deep breath and walked into the bathroom to take a look . . .

I WALK THE LINE

Now, we'd taken these tests before—a lot of them—but we never, ever saw "the blue line." Sure, we *thought* we saw the blue line. We squinted and held it up to lights and maybe sort of kind of *imagined* we saw the line. It's kind of like when you go bowling, and for some reason you think that after you throw a really crappy ball, if you just move your head a teeny bit to the left and look at the ball from another angle as it rolls down the alley and scream, "Get over! Get over!" it'll actually go that way. It's stupid, I know, but it's what all couples do when they don't get a positive test. You end up staring so hard at the little window that you're positive it's positive—but it isn't.

So once again we were all ready not to see the line. In fact, we were so ready that Julie decided to go back into the bathroom early to confirm our failure, while I volunteered to continue sitting on the couch watching TV. (No sense in both of us wasting our time, right?)

The next thing I know Julie comes bolting into the living room and collapses onto the floor screaming and crying, the pregnancy test clutched tightly in her hand. Being a guy, and thus relating all crying to bad things, I naturally expected the worst.

I was all set to utter those all-too-familiar words, "It's okay, sweetie, we can always try again . . ." when she triumphantly thrust the stick into the air like Arthur raising Excalibur and that's when I saw it—slowly materializing in that little plastic window, getting darker and darker, like some magical rune: *the blue line.* It didn't look like much, what with it being . . . well, a line that happens to be blue (after all, that *is* why they call it a blue line). But to us, it was the burning bush, the falling of the manna, the changing of water into wine, and every other miracle we could think of all rolled into one. It was a positive pregnancy test. Not just a positive, but a BFP—a "big fat positive!"

The next day we happily went to the clinic to take our beta test. When we got the call a few hours later, we were already riding the high from the (supposed) positive test on the HPT from the night before, but hearing it from the doctor's mouth made it real. I won't lie to you: After all those past failures, it felt pretty damn freakin' awesome!

After three unsuccessful tries, it finally worked. It was official. We were pregnant.

LOOK, HONEY! HE'S GOT MY EYES AND YOUR . . . VESTIGIAL TAIL?

What we as men have to realize is that an IVF pregnancy is much different from a regular pregnancy. I mean let's face it. It took a lot more than a cheap bottle of merlot on a Saturday night to get you both to this point, so it only makes sense that the pregnancy itself will be a lot more involved too.

For one thing, during those first couple of months of the pregnancy, your wife will be going in for ultrasounds—a whole lot of 'em. Every couple of weeks or so, in fact. That's normal. It's just to make sure the embryo is developing correctly.

Don't worry if you have no idea what you're seeing on the monitor. Until the doctor corrected me as to what part of the ultrasound I should be looking at, I was bursting with pride at having fathered my wife's spleen. Your fertility doctor will be able to tell you with some reasonable certainty that all systems are go. Plus, the little printouts make great mementos;

how many of us can say we have baby pictures from back when we looked like a cross between a tadpole and Winston Churchill?

I'M NOT PARANOID—IT'S JUST THAT EVERYONE IS OUT TO GET ME!!

Unfortunately, there's one thing I have to give you the heads-up about right now: From this point on, your wife will slowly devolve into a paranoid mess (albeit a beautiful one with that lovely pregnant glow). It's as inevitable as the talking-dog movie coming next summer to a theater near you.

But—and this is an *incredibly important* "but"—if there is one time in your marriage you absolutely, positively *must* cut her some slack, this is it. After going through such a trying experience (or two, or three, or six), she's keenly aware of her body. Every little hiccup, pain, cramp, bit of nausea— she'll be feeling it. And magnifying it. And then she'll race to her computer to access every medical database known to man, eventually concluding that she's suffering from whatever the worst possible scenario may be.

Relax. She's not crazy, and it's perfectly normal. Plus, there's really nothing you can do about it, short of completely canceling your Internet service—and I definitely wouldn't do that, because, and let's be perfectly frank here, the more pregnant and uncomfortable she gets, the more *you'll* be needing that Internet, if you catch my drift . . .

Much of the time, it comes down to how men and women

deal with problems. As I've said before, we men are, by nature, problem solvers. Generally, sitting around obsessing about problems, real or imagined, doesn't gibe with our mental wiring. If something's wrong, we fix it.

Women, on the other hand, sometimes dwell on problems just to dwell on problems. They're not necessarily looking for us to offer them solutions. They just want to be heard. This, of course, is completely insane and makes no sense to us, and is thus considered a problem in and of itself. And what do men do when faced with a problem? Everyone together now: "We must fix it!" But when your wife is pregnant, this rule goes right out the window, to be replaced with: "Just keep your mouth shut and get her whatever she wants." And life goes on . . .

GO AHEAD—MAKE YOUR MOVE

If you're like most couples going through fertility treatments, you've likely spent quite a bit of time at the bookstore (okay, well, at least your wife has). Even more likely is that you've frequented one special section. Most likely of all is that it's the section where you found this book.

Yep, I'm referring to none other than the dreaded "fertility" section. Your wife has probably spent hours and hours perusing the books here, a section usually placed in some dark, remote, cobwebbed area of the bookstore right next to the help desk, where employees just stare at you as you read, all the while shaking their heads sadly at your secret shame . . . Okay, fine, it's not really like that, but it sure can feel like it.

But guess what? All that's over now! That's right—go ahead and send the post office those change of address cards, baby—'cause you're moving!

Let me tell you, one of the most truly satisfying moments of a successful fertility treatment—you know, aside from that whole "you're finally pregnant" thing—is being able to stride proudly right past that dreaded fertility section to where they keep the books on *pregnancy.* It may not seem like a big deal, but let me tell you, it's huge.

(As a point of reference: Remember when you were a little kid and you watched *The Wizard of Oz* and everything at the beginning was that crappy brown color, and then the tornado comes and Dorothy's house lands on the witch and the midgets come out and everything's suddenly in so much color that it looks like a big bag of Skittles exploded? Yeah, well it's kind of like that. But better.)

Now your wife gets to skip happily to the books with names like *You're Pregnant!* and *Hey, You! Yeah, You! You're Pregnant!* and *Have Another Piece of Cake! Who Cares If People Think You're Fat?—You're Pregnant!*

From this point on, your big problem will consist of not having enough time to read fifteen different accounts of what type of produce to compare your child's size against for the next nine months. (Chick pea? Grape? Lima bean?)

But you know what? It's a freakin' *awesome* problem to have.

NOT A PROBLEM!

Emerging victorious from a fertility cycle leads to a few other situations I like to refer to as "the good problems":

- Anyone who knew you were doing IVF *has* to be told about the pregnancy—immediately. Forget about that old "we won't tell anyone until after the first trimester" saw. Think about it: It would be like your friend going on a date with the world's hottest supermodel and the next morning refusing to tell you what happened—a total dick move.

- Now instead of poring over fertility Web sites, your wife will be turning that obsession toward baby furniture catalogs and accessories Web sites. Look, I'll admit that up until this point I thought babies slept in simple wooden cribs and a stroller was just a car seat mounted on top of a shopping cart. Turns out there are co-sleepers and Moses baskets and glass vs. plastic bottles and organic vs. industrial and all sorts of decisions that you need to make. Wait. Scratch that. These are the decisions you *want* to make.

- How do you afford all of this crap after you've shelled out a small fortune on fertility treatments? Beats me. We're still trying to work that one out.

END OF THE LINE

So after all of this, you may be saying to yourself, "Wow! This sure sounds like a lot of hard work, for both my wife and me. Plus, even after going through all of that, there are still no guarantees! Wouldn't it just be easier to bail on the whole thing, take the money, and buy a boat or go to Hawaii or turn the basement into a cool game room with a pool table and vintage video games or something like that?"

Allow me put it to you this way: Think of the worst pain, either physical or emotional, that you've ever felt in your life. In fact, don't just think of it; try to really visualize it. Try to actually *feel* it again. You can't, right? The human body has this remarkable ability to forget pain. It's why women who have already given birth can go back and do it again. Sure, you may be able to remember the idea of the pain in an abstract way, but once the feeling is gone, it's gone.

The same idea applies to fertility treatments. Sure, it can be difficult. It can be discouraging. It may take more than a few tries. Hell, in our case it took four. But when it does finally happen, when the two of you look down at that strip of plastic and watch the little blue "positive" line slowly appear, everything you once thought was so impossible to get through will just feel like some faraway dream.

The most important thing to remember is that whatever happens, you're a team, and as hard as it seems right now, you will get through this. Just stay positive, keep a sense of humor about the process, and allow it to bring you closer together. After all, you're going to be a family now.

ALL JOKING ASIDE . . .

It took four attempts at IVF before it finally worked for Julie and me. Once we learned that the test was positive, we had regularly scheduled ultrasounds with our fertility doctor over the next several weeks. My work schedule didn't allow me to go to the first few, but one day I finally got the chance to come along.

Ask me if I ever had my doubts about fertility treatments. Ask me if I thought that at any time it would have been so much easier to give up. Ask me if I thought all of the hormones and pills and needles and sharps containers and doctor visits and yelling and screaming and crying and financial and emotional stress—basically three whole years of our life—was worth it.

If you had asked me any of those things at any other time during the process, I would have probably given you some very different answers.

But as I sat in that darkened exam room and looked into the ultrasound monitor, I watched my son's little heart beating, his tiny arms and legs moving around. Then I looked up into Julie's beautiful face, and for the first time saw not just my wife, but the mother of my children. And it finally hit me: We had done it. This was *our* family.

And I thought to myself, "Oh yeah. It was all worth it."

AFTERWORD

AKA "Post-Partum Impressions"

On March 21, 2009, at 4:21 PM, Connor Joseph Wolfe came into the world, and more importantly, into Julie's and my life. As I watched the nurse put him down on the sterile table in the delivery room to clean him off, I saw him for the first time: He was small, wrinkled, semibald, and dripping with blood and mucus. In other words, he was *gorgeous*.

As I held him, it was hard to believe that the long, painful road that Julie and I had to travel in order to get to this point was over. All of the frustration, the anger, the doctors, the shots, the disappointments—they all seemed to disappear from our memories, only to be replaced with . . . this baby. Our son. Of course the long, painful road of parenthood was just beginning, but at least for that moment, we could rest.

I wanted to write this part of the book not so much to gloat (although, yes, that does seem to be a good enough reason), but to give other would-be fathers hope. Believe me, after the first three tries at IVF, I wasn't expecting the fourth to work any more than I'd expect the next *Indiana Jones* movie to have a coherent plot. But it did—the fertility treatment, I mean (jury's still out on Dr. Jones)—and for that I am eternally grateful. Grateful not just to our doctor who finally made it happen, but also to the doctor who couldn't the previous three times. It was due to these failures that our second doctor was able to pinpoint the problem and *KAPOW*! Heeeere's Connor!

It might sound like a dopey, new age bullshit thing to say, but if there's one guiding principle I have found that seems to govern my life, it's that everything happens for a reason. Sure, I may not know what that reason may be until days, weeks, even years later, but when I look back on the story of my life, I see things interconnecting and working out in ways that are, well, nothing less than amazing.

In this case, when I found out that I was going to have problems conceiving a child, I felt like I was the lowest piece of crap in the world. And yes, there are obviously already a lot of pretty low pieces of crap in the world, so that put me really, really far down there on the crap scale. Now, it took a few years for things to finally work out, but it occurs to me that if things hadn't happened in the exact way they happened—the failures, our hopes rising and rising, only to be dashed back to the ground—well, who knows if we would have Connor. Yes, we may have achieved our goal of having a child eventually, but he absolutely would not have been Connor. At least not the Connor that we have now. I know you don't know him (and really, it's too small of an apartment to invite everyone in), but if you could see him, and witness the joy in his eyes and hear his happy little squeal every morning when we come in to wake him up . . . well, you'd know what I mean.

Yeah, yeah, I know I'm being mushy, but truthfully, it didn't seem like it was possible to love something as much as we love him. At this point, though, I'm pretty convinced that everything's possible, given an opportunity.

———

When I was younger, I was always curious about whether or not having a family would change me too much. Well, I don't know if I've changed so much as circumstances have. I mean, things are definitely different now that I've been assimilated into the great "Fatherhood Collective": Dirty martinis have been replaced by dirty diapers, breasts have taken on a much more utilitarian function than I ever dreamed they could, and for some reason I can't seem to listen to *Cat's in the Cradle* by Harry Chapin anymore without getting all misty eyed. (It's just so damn *sad* that the son turned out to be just like his father at the end . . . God, that always gets me!)

Do I feel like a dad? Truthfully, no, I don't. I always thought that when I had a kid I'd become wise and all knowing, and maybe suddenly have a yearning to go out and putter around the yard and swear a lot when the utility bill arrived. As it turns out, that doesn't really happen.

I mean, sure, this year I finally got a Fathers' Day card—a real one, not just one from the cats. And I get to say "my son" a lot, even if I don't really have to. And sometimes I just sit and stare at Connor and really find myself looking forward to playing with him as he gets older, watching sports with him on Sunday afternoons, arguing over who would win in a fight between Superman and Hercules (I gotta give it to Supes on that one. He could just throw Hercules into the sun), and all those fun father/son things.

But then I remember how I'm also going to have to do the hard stuff: punish him when he misbehaves, get down on him when he doesn't do his best in school, teach him how to treat a woman, maybe even have "the talk." (I'm actually quite curious to see how that one plays out—hey, he might feel more comfortable talking to his mother about that sort of stuff.) All part of being a dad, I suppose.

Oh, who am I kidding? Actually, I'm excited about the whole thing. This is what I've wanted my whole life, and now, thanks to the miracles of modern technology, I have it. Truth be told, I'm already kind of thinking ahead to the next kid. You know, another IVF to round the family out with a little girl. I figure I'll broach the subject with Julie in another few months.

Well, maybe in a couple of years. For some reason she seems really worn out . . .

ACKNOWLEDGMENTS

This book would not have been possible without the help of so many, many people, chief among whom is my agent, Sarah Jane Freymann, who had faith that a simple little proposal with a smutty-sounding title had what it took to become a fully realized book with a smutty-sounding title.

Also a huge thanks goes out to my editor at HarperCollins, Gabe Robinson, whose skill and infinite patience truly brought out the best in my writing—despite my chronic "its" vs. "it's" problem. (Sorry, Gabe. Really, I'm a teacher. I should know better!)

Another big thank you to Jessica Sinsheimer; but for her gumption, I wouldn't be able to write these acknowledgements.

To my parents, Stan and Dorene: For all you've done for me throughout my life, a simple "thank you" seems woefully inadequate, but I offer one up all the same.

Also my love and appreciation to my mother-in-law, Phyllis, and to my father-in-law, Jerry, a man I'm absolutely sure was—and still is—looking out for us from that big Union Hall in the sky.

And while I'm on the subject of divine aid, thank you God for making sure everything ended up happening in the right place and at the right time. I truly enjoy your work!

To our family and friends who stood by us throughout our years of struggles, your support means more than I can express.

A special, never-before-attempted-in-print "dual mega–thank you" to both Dr. Michael Vermesh and Dr. Eliran Mor, two of the finest reproductive endocrinologists a couple could ask for. What can I say? The two of you are miracle workers who made our dreams come true.

And finally, to my wife, Julie: Even though it wasn't your intention to be "research" for a book, I literally couldn't have done this without you, and I love you.

GLOSSARY

Your (Nearly) Complete
Infertility-to-English Dictionary

This book has presented you with a lot of facts. Obviously, you won't remember all of them. Or most of them. Hell, you should be happy if you remembered where it was on the bookshelf. Don't feel bad, though. If you did know all this stuff, you probably didn't need the book to begin with, and if you are one of those guys—good for you. Want a cookie?

For the rest of us, a glossary of terms is always a good thing to have, because believe me, your wife is going to be throwing around a lot of strange words, abbreviations, acronyms. Hell, you should see the glossaries in her books. Now by no means is this a complete glossary. Half the things I don't understand! But, in the spirit of your old high school cheat sheets—c'mon, no way you got that A in European Lit. legit!—I'm pleased to share some of the more common things you'll need to know.

Really, feel free to show off to her exactly how much you know now. She'll think you're awesome! Well, at least until the hormones start to kick in . . .

A

agonist—A drug or chemical that produces a particular reaction in the body, often mimicking a naturally occurring substance. Think of it as a drug sporting a really good fake ID.

amniotic sac—A membrane filled with fluid (called, appropriately enough, amniotic fluid), in which the fetus is suspended.

aspiration—The process of using a needle to remove the egg cell from an ovarian follicle during the retrieval portion of an IVF cycle. Don't worry. Your wife'll be heavily sedated.

aspiration cycle—ART cycle in which one or more follicles are opened up in order to get at the egg cells inside.

assisted hatching—A procedure in IVF done right before transfer where a lab technician pierces the zona (outer membrane) of the egg with a drop of acid in the hopes that the embryo inside will then separate from the egg and implant in the uterus. It looks better than it reads.

assisted reproductive technology (ART)—Everything inclusive of the in vitro treatments utilized to get your wife pregnant, including in vitro fertilization, embryo transfers, gamete intrafallopian transfer (see GIFT), zygote intrafallopian transfer (see ZIFT), surrogates, and egg and embryo donations.

B

baby aspirin—Your wife is told to take it as a blood thinner. Really. Don't think she has a problem.

beta hCG test (also β-hCG)—A test that measures the amount of hCG in the blood, which is an indicator of whether or not your wife is pregnant.

BFN—An abbreviation used by your wife and her "Internet friends" all too often on the fertility discussion boards. It means a "big fat negative" result on a home pregnancy test (HPT). We don't like them.

BFP—On the other hand, the "big fat positive" is what you want to see.

blastocyst—An embryo developing normally by day five or six after fertilization. Once again, has nothing to do with explosives, so calm down if your doctor tells you he sees one. It's good.

C

controlled ovarian hyperstimulation (COH)—Using hormones to cause the development of multiple ovarian follicles in order to obtain multiple eggs.

corpus luteum—The mass of cells that are left over after the release of an egg from a follicle during ovulation.

Responsible for the production of progesterone, they are absolutely necessary in order to keep a pregnancy viable.

cryopreservation—The freezing and storage of gametes, zygotes, or embryos for use in a later cycle, or possibly for use as donor embryos, a.k.a. "the Walt Disney." (Okay, they don't call it that. They should, but they don't.)

E

embryo—Your baby from the time of fertilization to the end of the eighth week after fertilization. Not nearly as cute as you'd hope, but it should be later on.

embryo donation—The transfer from a donor of an embryo that did not genetically originate from either the recipient (your wife) or you (you).

embryo transfer (ET)—This is also known as "your kid's first big trip." The IVF procedure by which three- or five-day-old embryos are taken from the petri dishes and inserted into your wife's waiting womb. Oddly enough, when your baby is born he or she will bear a striking resemblance to the lovable alien E.T. Coincidence? Yeah, probably.

endometriosis—A condition in which endometrium grows outside of the uterus. It can grow anywhere in the body, and it bleeds monthly as well, no matter where it is. And yes, it's weird.

endometrium—The tissue that lines the uterus and is shed every month during a woman's menstruation.

ethyl oleate—A thinner, more "liquidy" substitute for the thick oil medium that makes up the bulk of most progester-one shots, and therefore, a lot less painful to your loved one's posterior.

F

fertilization—When the sperm penetrates the egg cell and results in the formation and development of a zygote.

fetus—The technical term for your baby from eight weeks after fertilization until birth, at which point it officially becomes a "deduction."

FMU—Another one of those annoying fertility Web site acronyms, meaning "first morning urine"—the preferred urine for home pregnancy tests since that's when the concentration of hCG is highest.

follicular cyst—The most common type of ovarian cyst—basically an egg follicle that grows too big, balloons up, and explodes when ovulation doesn't occur. It hurts, but is generally not too dangerous.

Follistim—A recombinant gonadotropin containing highly purified FSH, oftentimes used during IVF, derived from Chinese hamster ovarian cells.

FSH (follicle stimulating hormone)—The hormone that causes an immature follicle to produce an egg.

full-term birth—A birth that takes place at thirty-seven or more completed weeks of gestational age. Another one of those "you want this" terms.

G

gamete intrafallopian transfer (GIFT)—ART procedure in which both male and female sex cells (sperm and eggs) are transferred to the fallopian tubes in the hopes they'll meet and fertilize by the time they make it down to the uterus. Like a jet fighter refueling in midair.

gestational age—The "true" age of an embryo or fetus calculated by adding fourteen days (two weeks) to the number of completed weeks since fertilization. Never ask a fetus for this age though. It's considered rude.

gestational carrier (surrogate)—A woman in whom a pregnancy results from fertilization with third-party sperm and eggs, and who agrees to the pregnancy under a contract that states that the baby will go to one or both of the persons producing the sex cells. Sometimes the stuff Lifetime movies are made of.

gestational sac—A precursor to the amniotic sac, it's a fluid-filled structure containing an embryo, and it develops early in pregnancy. It's usually the only thing you can see in an ultrasound before the fetus is identified.

GIFT—See gamete intrafallopian transfer.

gonadotropins—Hormones secreted by the pituitary gland, primarily FSH, LH, and hCG.

H

hCG (human chorionic gonadotropin)—1) the IVF "trigger shot" that, once injected, causes ovulation within thirty-six to forty-eight hours, 2) a hormone made by the human embryo that helps sustain the corpus luteum, which, in turn, produces the progesterone needed to keep the uterus a nice, comfy place for baby, 3) the hormone your doctor will be looking for when he or she tests your blood for signs of pregnancy. That's a lot of definitions for three little letters!

host uterus—See gestational carrier.

HPT—Home pregnancy test, a.k.a. "the pee stick."

I

ICSI (intracytoplasmic sperm injection)—A really cool and highly advanced technique in which a single sperm cell is injected into an egg before the fertilized egg is transferred back to the woman's body, primarily utilized in cases of male-factor infertility. Did I mention it was cool?

implantation—Five to seven days after fertilization when the blastocyst attaches to and penetrates the endometrium.

infertility—The official term used to describe the situation after failure to have a live birth after trying (you know, "really *trying*") for one year.

IVF (in vitro fertilization)—Where embryo fertilization happens outside the uterus (as opposed to in vivo fertilization, where it happens inside the uterus). Better spawning through chemistry.

L

LH (luteinizing hormone)—A hormone that stimulates ovulation and the development of the corpus luteum.

live birth rate—A really important number when considering a particular fertility clinic or doctor, made up of the percentage of all of the cycles that lead to a live birth.

Lupron—An agonist hormone used to suppress the pituitary gland and prevent premature ovulation. Taken as a subcutaneous injection, it decreases normal levels of both FSH and LH. Sneaky thing!

M

Menopur—A medication containing both FSH and LH, used to stimulate egg follicle growth and maturation. Based on the urine of menopausal women. Eww.

micromanipulation (also referred to as assisted fertilization)—The use of special technology that allows operative procedures to be performed on the oocyte, sperm, or embryo, like ICSI, PGD, or GIFT.

microscopic epididymal sperm aspiration (MESA)—A procedure in which sperm cells are obtained directly from within the testes, often not in the most pleasant manner (there are needles involved).

miscarriage—Losing a pregnancy before twenty weeks of gestation.

O

oocyte donation—A donation of egg cells (oocytes) from a third party, i.e., an egg donor.

P

PCOS—See polycystic ovarian syndrome.

pessaries—Vaginal suppositories. Progesterone and estrogen given as luteal phase support during IVF and administered in the form of capsules or tablets inserted vaginally. Messy.

PGD—See preimplantation genetic diagnosis.

PIO (progesterone in oil)—A really thick, oily concoction of progesterone injected intramuscularly (as in her butt) to help thicken the uterine lining after embryos have been transferred. Because both the administration of LH and the physical retrieval of eggs interferes with natural progesterone production, supplemental progesterone is typically given during IVF until twelve weeks or so into a successful pregnancy. Doesn't hurt as much as it looks like it should, though the bruising can get pretty spectacular.

POAS—More fun with crazy discussion board acronyms—"pee on a stick"—i.e., to take an HPT. See why we guys don't join these chat groups?

polycystic ovarian syndrome (PCOS)—A disorder due to hormone fluctuations in which LH levels are high while FSH levels remain low. This results in ovarian follicles that are unable to release their eggs and, as a result, often develop into fluid-filled cysts.

preclinical pregnancy (biochemical pregnancy)—Saying that you're pregnant based only on the traces of biochemicals found in urine or blood tests, before an ultrasound actually detects physical proof.

preimplantation genetic diagnosis (PGD)—Taking a sample of cells from preimplantation embryos in order to check for genetic and/or chromosomal disorders.

prenatal vitamins—Vitamins specially formulated to support healthy pregnancy. Your wife will go crazy trying to remember if she took them each day.

progesterone—Female hormones released during ovulation responsible for preparing the uterus for implantation. Also, a really big ugly shot you need to give your wife for a few weeks toward the end of an IVF cycle in order to increase the natural progesterone in her system and get her uterus sticky enough to accept the embryo.

R

RE—See reproductive endocrinologist.

recipient—Refers to a woman who receives a donor egg or embryo from another woman.

recombinant gonadotropins—Gonadotropins containing only FSH that are created by injecting the DNA of a particular human gonadotropin into Chinese hamster ovarian cells, which then replicate into the new gonadotropin. Wild, huh?

reproductive endocrinologist—The technical title for what we call a fertility doctor. Sure it may cost more to print it on a business card, but I think it's worth it.

retrieval—The procedure in which a long needle is inserted through the vaginal wall and into the ovaries, where individual follicles are harvested for eggs. The eggs are then fertilized with sperm. Since your doctor wants to limit the screaming, this is usually performed while the patient is under general anesthesia.

S

surrogate mother—See gestational carrier.

T

testicular sperm extraction (TESE)—Procedure in which sperm are obtained directly from the testicle, by either aspiration or surgical excision of testicular tissue. Ow.

transfer—See embryo transfer.

trigger shot—The intramuscular injection of hCG given to trigger ovulation thirty-six to forty-eight hours before retrieval.

U

ultrasound (sometimes abbreviated as US)—A medical imaging technique used to visualize internal organs. In IVF, the vaginal ultrasound is typically used to get the probe closer to the uterus and ovaries. The probe is mounted on a long wand that is inserted into the vagina and moved around. Yes, it's as embarrassingly intimate as it sounds.

urinary gonadotropins—Gonadotropins containing both LH and FSH extracted from the highly purified urine of post-menopausal women (a.k.a. "that one made from old lady pee").

Z

zona—The thick membrane covering the female egg that the male sperm normally has to break through in order to start the fertilization process. In the process of assisted hatching, a lab tech makes a small hole in it in the hopes of increasing the chances of the developing embryo implanting in the uterus after transfer.

zygote—The cell that results from your sperm and her egg making whoopee and fertilizing.

zygote intrafallopian transfer (ZIFT)—Procedure in which the zygote is transferred directly into the fallopian tube in the hopes that it will then travel down and implant in the uterus.

ENDNOTES

a   Chandra et al., *Fertility, family planning, and reproductive health of U.S. women: Data from the 2002 National Survey of Family Growth*, National Center for Health Statistics, Vital Health Stat. 23 (25), 2005.

b   Chandra et al., *Fertility, family planning, and reproductive health of U.S. women: Data from the 2002 National Survey of Family Growth*, National Center for Health Statistics, Vital Health Stat. 23 (25), 2005.

c   *American Society for Reproductive Medicine*. American Society for Reproductive Medicine (www.asrm.org/Patients/faqs.html#Q2), September 28, 2009.

d   Endometriosis Research Center, Frequently Asked Questions (www.endocenter.org/endofaq.htm), July 17, 2009.

e   World Health Organization, *WHO Laboratory Manual for the Examination of Human Semen and Semen-Cervical Mucus Interaction*, 3rd ed. (Cambridge: Cambridge University Press, 1992).

f   Jay Mechling, "Gun Play is NOT Bad for Boys," *American Journal of Play*, Vol. 1., no. 2 (2008).

INDEX